Stop Worrying About Cholesterol!

Better Ways to Avoid a Heart Attack and Get Healthy

Richard E. Tapert, D.O.

ISBN 0-7414-2455-X

Disclaimer: This book is not intended as a substitute for medical diagnosis or treatment. All potentially serious health problems must be managed by a trained physician.

Published by:

INFINITY
PUBLISHING.COM

1094 New DeHaven Street, Suite 100
West Conshohocken, PA 19428-2713
Info@buybooksontheweb.com
www.buybooksontheweb.com
Toll-free (877) BUY BOOK
Local Phone (610) 941-9999
Fax (610) 941-9959

Printed in the United States of America

Printed on Recycled Paper

Published March 2005

Dedication

To Karen, my devoted wife, without whose numerous suggestions, countless hours of proof reading, and inspiration, this book would not have been possible.

Table of Contents

Part II: What Really Matters?

Introduction

• You've been told that cholesterol is something to be feared. That cholesterol is the enemy. That when you eat it, it will build up in your arteries and eventually cause heart disease, heart attacks, and early death.

• You've been bombarded on television and in popular magazines by ads which encourage you to ask your doctor to prescribe the latest cholesterol lowering drug, and given the message that the lower the level of cholesterol in your blood, the less likely you will be to have a heart attack, stroke, or other circulation disaster.

• You've been told by the advertising media to avoid eggs, eat "Egg Beaters". You've been told to avoid butter and lard, and to use various types of margarine, "Crisco", and other fake fats. All of this to avoid the devious, sneaky enemy, **CHOLESTEROL!**

• Perhaps you're taking one of the expensive cholesterol lowering drugs known as statins, and returning to your doctor periodically for blood tests to see if your liver, kidneys, or muscles have been damaged by the drug. Or perhaps you are experiencing confusion, memory problems, weakness, excessive fatigue, or muscle pain, (increasingly common side effects of the statin drugs) and beginning to wonder if it all makes sense.

The truth about cholesterol!

• My mission is to teach you the truth about cholesterol and its alleged relationship to heart disease. You will learn that cholesterol is not the enemy, that it is not the cause of heart attacks. You will learn the many very important roles that cholesterol plays in your body. You will learn that the real dangerous fats are the ones that you have been "brain-washed" into eating if you have been following the advice of the food industry, the medical establishment, and the popular media.

• You will learn that the early research designed to prove the diet/cholesterol/heart disease connection actually proved that there was no connection between dietary cholesterol and heart disease, and that voluminous research since then has also verified that the cholesterol that you eat has no causative role in heart disease.

• You will learn that the animal foods your grand-parents ate on the farm a few generations ago, when combined with lots of vegetables and fruits, provide the healthy fats and other important nutrients that you and your arteries need to keep you functioning to a ripe old age. You will also learn about other important "good fats" that will actually prevent and treat many of the common ailments that plague us through the aging process.

• And we will explore the fact that the low-fat food propaganda from the processed food industry over the last thirty years has been a major contributor to our current epidemic of obesity and adult-onset diabetes. Now teenagers and even preteens are developing "adult-onset diabetes."

• You will learn of the serious dangers inherent in taking the commonly over-prescribed statin drugs. You will learn of the science that exposes the real causes of heart disease. And, most importantly, you will learn what you need to know to avoid heart attacks, and live a long healthy life.

Have you been lied to? Lied to by the medical establishment? Lied to by the food industry? Lied to by the media?

In this book I will help you sort out the truth from the commercially motivated lies. I will provide you with numerous sources to check so that you can verify the facts which I present. I will direct you to the foods and nutritional supplements that will help you achieve optimal health. And, should you need a doctor or a nutritionist, I will help you find health practitioners who utilize healthy alternative methods of preventing and treating heart disease and other diseases of aging. The rest will be up to you.

My hope is that you will realize that often the truth is something you must search for. In this most important and vital area of heart health I aim to help you find the truth.

Yes, you can stop worrying about cholesterol, avoid heart attacks, and live a long healthy life!

Part I

Cholesterol! Does It Matter?

In questions of science, the authority of a thousand is not worth the humble reasoning of a single individual. **Galileo**

Chapter One

The Lipid Hypothesis

Four important questions:

Does the animal fat and cholesterol you eat cause elevation of your blood cholesterol level?

Does the animal fat and cholesterol you eat cause heart disease?

Does the cholesterol in your blood cause heart disease?

Does lowering your cholesterol prevent you from having heart attacks?

The idea that fat and cholesterol consumption is the reason for our current epidemic of heart disease originated early in the twentieth century when it was observed that the plaques in the arteries of heart attack victims contained fat and cholesterol. The Framingham study, which began in 1948 and continued for many years, was designed to prove "the lipid hypothesis". The lipid hypothesis is simply the theory that there is a direct relationship between the amount of saturated fat (animal fat) and cholesterol in the diet, and the incidence of coronary heart disease (heart attacks).

The Framingham Study is used by those who endorse the lipid hypothesis, as proof of the validity of the lipid hypothesis. In this study approximately 5000 people were followed and studied every five years. There were two groups. Those who consumed large amounts of animal fat and cholesterol were compared with those who consumed very little. Forty years after the start of this study, its director, Dr. William Castelli, reluctantly admitted, *In Framingham, Massachusetts the more saturated fat one ate, the more cholesterol one ate, the more calories one ate, the lower the person's serum cholesterol. We found that the people who ate the most cholesterol, ate the most saturated fat, and ate the most calories, weighed the least and were the most active.* Yes, those who ate the most cholesterol and fat gained the least amount of weight. Although the study did find an association between high levels of blood cholesterol and increased likelihood of future heart attacks, the elevated cholesterol was only one of over 240 "risk factors" that were associated with increased risk of heart attacks. And this association was found only in young and middle aged men. **In the 30 year follow-up of the Framingham Study, high cholesterol was not predictive of heart attack at all after the age of 47. In other words, according to the Framingham Study, once a man reaches the age of 48 there is no relationship between high levels of cholesterol and dying of a heart attack.** And most alarming is the fact that those whose cholesterol dropped without any intervention ran a much higher risk of a heart attack than those whose cholesterol increased. The **significantly increased** risk of dying from heart disease and from other diseases in those whose cholesterol **decreased** is so contrary to what we have been led to believe that I feel it is important to print the whole abstract of the article that points out that fact.

This article appeared in the prestigious Journal of the American Medical Association on April 24, 1987 under the title, **Cholesterol and mortality. Thirty years of follow-up from the Framingham study.** Its authors are the chief investigators of the Framingham study, W.P. Castelli, K.M. Anderson, and D. Levy. Here is the abstract: *From 1951 to 1955 serum cholesterol levels were measured in 1959 men and 2415 women aged between 31 and 65 years who were free of cardiovascular disease (CVD) and cancer. Under age 50 years cholesterol levels are directly related with 30 year overall and CVD mortality; overall death increases 5% and CVD death 9% for each 10 mg/dL. After age 50 years there is no increased overall mortality with either high or low serum cholesterol levels. There is a direct association between <u>falling</u> cholesterol levels over the first 14 years and mortality over the following 18 years (11% overall and 14% CVD death rate <u>increase</u> per 1mg/dL per year drop in cholesterol levels). Under age 50 years these data suggest that having a very low cholesterol level improves longevity. After age 50 years the association of mortality with cholesterol values is confounded by people whose cholesterol levels are falling—perhaps due to diseases predisposing to death.*

Yes, those whose cholesterol <u>dropped</u> had a significantly <u>increased</u> risk of dying!

And yet, the American Heart Association and the National Heart, Lung, and Blood Institute issued the following statement: *The results of the Framingham study indicate that a 1% reduction... of cholesterol (corresponds to a) 2% reduction in coronary heart disease risk.*

How do we account for that? The authors of the study said that for every 1% drop in cholesterol level there was an **increase** of 14% in cardiovascular deaths, and yet the AHA and the NHLBI released a statement that 1% reduction of cholesterol corresponds to a 2% **reduction** in coronary heart disease risk.

In studies of women and of men and women who already have had a heart attack, high cholesterol has little predictive power, if any at all. And yet, the entire population has been taught to fear cholesterol. Most importantly, the public health authorities, who were looking for proof of the lipid hypothesis, confused **statistical association** with **causation**. The Framingham Study did not prove the lipid hypothesis. It actually was one of many studies that began to disprove the hypothesis.

However, by the time the Framingham Study was well underway, the commercial interests that were to enormously benefit from the development and sale of the artificially modified fats, the margarines and vegetable oils, had gained a major foothold in the marketplace, convincing the public that the proof was in, and that it is time to start avoiding animal fats such as butter, dairy products, beef, poultry, and eggs, and to use margarine, vegetable oils and synthetic shortenings. As we shall see, this was a major turning point in the deterioration of the health of the American people, a deterioration that also spread to the rest of the civilized world.

But haven't there been many studies that support the diet/cholesterol/heart disease connection? What about all the scientific studies performed by respected, highly qualified researchers, and sponsored by government agencies, major drug companies, and big powerful organizations like the American Heart Association and the National Heart, Lung, and Blood Institute? Isn't there a consensus among these experts that lowering cholesterol by diet and/or drugs will help us to avoid heart attacks and live longer? How could all these experts be wrong? The answer to this question is not a simple one. To the reader who generally regards medical science as being honest, uncorrupted, and dedicated to the

10

improvement of mankind's health, it is time to take a long hard look at the facts. In matters of such importance to your health and longevity you must look beyond what you are being told by most doctors, and beyond the slick, high-powered media ads that the multi-billion dollar drug industry is putting before you with ever increasing frequency.

The facts are that many of the studies that are quoted to promote the diet/cholesterol/heart disease connection were poorly designed and poorly conducted. Many did not produce the results that have been claimed for them. Many have been quoted in misleading ways. When the studies showed some favorable effect from lowering cholesterol, the effect was exaggerated, often by manipulating statistics. And very importantly, many other studies seriously question or actually contradict the mainstream diet/cholesterol/heart disease consensus. These studies, the ones that do not support the mainstream view, are not acknowledged or quoted. This is called selective citation. And this process is the foundation upon which one of the biggest deceptions in medical history has been perpetrated on an unsuspecting public.

A detailed analysis and criticism of all the studies is a very complex process, and it makes for tedious and difficult reading. But for those who have serious interest in the matter, I highly recommend *The Cholesterol Myths: Exposing the Fallacy that Saturated Fat and Cholesterol Cause Heart Disease*, an excellent and thoroughly documented book by Uffe Ravnskov, M.D. Ravnskov is a most outstanding physician and researcher. A graduate of the University of Copenhagen, he worked as a physician for 17 years in the fields of surgery, radiology, neurology, pediatrics, and internal medicine. He has published over 40 scientific studies on blood lipids (fats), and about 20 on inflammatory kidney disease. In *The Cholesterol Myths*, he expertly analyzes the studies that purport to prove the lipid hypothesis and points out the statistical manipulations, the sloppy research, the bias, the exaggerations of favorable results and the ignoring of massive amounts of contradictory findings.

A study published in Lancet, one of the world's most respected medical journals, in 1983 involved several thousand men. Half were told to reduce saturated fat and cholesterol (animal fat) and to stop smoking and to increase the amounts of unsaturated oils such as vegetable oils and margarines. The others were to continue eating as much animal fat and cholesterol as they desired and were not advised to quit smoking. After one year, those who were on the so-called "good diet" with lots of margarine and vegetable oils had twice as many deaths than those on the so-called "bad diet" in spite of the fact that those on the "bad diet" continued to smoke.

Numerous population studies have demonstrated that people who consume animal fats, such as butter, lard, meat, eggs, and dairy products have significantly lower incidence of heart disease than those who have adopted the "modern" substitutions (margarine, shortening, etc.). Examples: A study comparing Yemenite Jews living in Yemen where they consumed animal fats, to Yemenite Jews living in Israel who consumed margarine and vegetable fats, found that those who consumed the animal fats had a very low incidence of diabetes and heart disease. Those who were consuming the margarine and vegetable fats had a very high incidence of the same diseases. (The Israeli Yemenites, those who ate lots of margarine and vegetable oils and suffered much heart disease were also documented to be consuming large amounts of sugar. We will discuss the role of refined sugar in the causation of heart disease in a later chapter.)

A study comparing people living in northern India who consume 17 times more animal fat than those living in southern India found that those in the north have 7 times less coronary heart disease.

Eskimos, who in their native habitat consume large amounts of animal fat in the form of fish and other marine animals, are remarkably healthy, vigorous, and free of disease.

If heart attacks are caused by eating too much animal fat, heart attacks should increase when animal fat consumption goes up and should decrease when animal fat consumption goes down. Let's take a look at what has actually happened when major changes in animal fat consumption have occurred.

In the United States heart disease mortality increased by about 10 times between 1930 and 1960. During that thirty year period animal fat consumption decreased significantly.

In England heart attacks increased about 10 times between 1930 and 1970, while animal fat consumption has neither increased nor decreased since 1910.

In Yugoslavia, between 1955 and 1965 animal fat consumption decreased 25%. Heart attack deaths increased 3 to 4 times during that same decade.

In the Framingham study, during the decline of animal fat consumption, non-fatal heart attacks increased, but fatal heart attacks decreased. Although the promoters of the lipid hypothesis proposed a convoluted explanation for this peculiarity, the logical explanation is that treatment for heart attack victims improved significantly during the same time period.

In Japan, from 1950 to 1970, while animal fat consumption increased, fatal heart attacks also increased. This would seem to support the diet/cholesterol/heart disease theory. However, closer analysis reveals that the increase only occurred in people over the age of 70, and particularly over the age of 80. The younger people died <u>less</u> often of heart disease in spite of consuming <u>more</u> animal fat. The explanation is that, after World War II, general health of the Japanese people had improved to the extent that many more survived to old age, and were thus more likely to die of heart disease, since it is a disease of old age. What has happened since 1970? Consumption of animal fat has continued to increase. Yet, contrary to predictions from the lipid hypothesis promoters, fatal heart attacks have decreased in all age groups.

In Switzerland, after World War II heart disease deaths decreased while animal fat consumption increased by 20%.

During the 1960s Dr. George Mann made a study of the Masai people in Kenya. These are slender people who in their native environment are generally very active, doing much walking and running to tend their cattle. Their diet is extreme. They live entirely on milk, blood, and meat. Lots of cholesterol and saturated fat! According to Dr. Mann they drink over one half gallon of high fat milk per day, which includes about one half a pound of butterfat. This is in addition to large amounts of meat. It is reported that at parties, consumption of 4 to 10 pounds of meat per person is not unusual. One would expect that, if the diet/cholesterol/heart disease theory were correct, there would be epidemic levels of heart attack deaths. But Dr. Mann found that, not only did they not die of heart disease, but their blood cholesterol levels were extremely low, lower by about 50% than the levels of most Americans. On studying the post-mortem hearts and aortas of the Masai, it was found that atherosclerosis was present, but myocardial infarction (heart attack) had not occurred in any of them.

What happens to the blood cholesterol levels of the Masai if they move from their native environment, and consume a lower fat diet? A study was done by Jose Day, M.D. of St. Mary's Hospital London. Twenty-six Masai men who had relocated to the city of Nairobi were studied. In Nairobi they had many more food choices, thus, the amount of animal fat in their diet was much lower than that of their kinsmen living in their native habitat. It would be expected that their cholesterol levels would be lower, since they were consuming less fat. However, their blood cholesterol levels were 25% higher than that of their counterparts living on the extremely high fat diet.

The bottom line here is that one can consume high levels of animal fat and have normal, or even low, blood cholesterol levels.

These studies and many others that do not support the diet/cholesterol/heart disease connection are simply ignored. They are simply not cited in the literature by those who have a vested interest in maintaining the status quo, in increasing the consumption of artificially modified fats, and bolstering the multi-billion dollar cholesterol-lowering drug industry.

Most of the studies that have shown, through diet modification or drug therapy, a slight reduction in coronary heart disease or coronary heart disease deaths have also shown an increase in overall mortality. Thus, substituting processed vegetable fat for animal fat and taking cholesterol lowering drugs resulted in more deaths from cancer, brain hemorrhage, suicide and violent death.

This was the case in the study called The Lipid Research Clinics Coronary Primary Prevention Trial. All participants were given a low-cholesterol, low-saturated fat diet, and some were also given a cholesterol lowering drug. Those given a cholesterol lowering drug had a reduced rate of coronary artery disease, according to the researchers, although independent researchers who evaluated the data found that there was no significant difference in the coronary disease rate between the two groups. There was, however, an increase in deaths from stroke, cancer, and suicide. A significant difference in any study result means that the difference is beyond what would occur by chance.

The famous heart surgeon, Michael DeBakey, M.D. was one of many who have observed that the level of cholesterol in the blood does not correlate with the incidence of heart disease.

His study of 1700 patients, which was published in the Journal of the American Medical Association, found no relationship between the level of cholesterol in the blood and the incidence of atherosclerosis (hardening of the arteries). Those who had low cholesterol had as much atherosclerosis as those with high cholesterol. It is well established that half of all heart attacks occur in people who have normal or low cholesterol.

With statistics you can change black to white. Thus said Dr. Ravnskov in his brilliant analysis of some of the statistical manipulation that has been extensively utilized by those "experts" who have defined and promoted the diet/cholesterol/heart disease connection. The MRFIT (Multiple Risk Factor Intervention Trial) is considered one of the greatest medical experiments in history. Blood cholesterol was measured in approximately 360,000 American middle-aged men. Of those, 1200 were selected for the intervention studies. There were also a large number of studies done on the over 300,000 "screenees" who for various reasons were excluded from the intervention study. The screenees were divided into 10 groups (deciles) according to their cholesterol values. The first decile consisted of the men with the lowest cholesterol values, and the tenth decile consisted of those with the highest values. After 6 years the number of deaths due to heart attack in each decile were compared. According to Dr. Jeremiah Stamler, director of the study, the risk of dying from a heart attack with cholesterol above 265 was 413% higher than with cholesterol below 170. Sounds alarming! But let's look at the actual figures. Four hundred ninety four of those with the highest cholesterol (10th decile) had died of a heart attack. That is 1.3% of the total number of men in that group. (98.7% of the group with the highest cholesterol were still alive.) Among those with the lowest cholesterol (1st decile) ninety-five or 0.3% had died. (99.7% survived). Thus the difference in number of deaths between the highest cholesterol group and the lowest was only one percentage point (1.3% minus 0.3%). One percentage point does not sound nearly as alarming as 413%. But, yes, it is true that 1.3 is 413% of 0.3. So we see one of the many ways that statistics can be manipulated to exaggerate and create a more impressive or alarming response.

But a more important point is that the tenth decile (the highest cholesterol group) contained individuals who suffer with the rare inherited disease called "familial hyper-cholesterolemia." This condition, which affects a little less than 1% of human beings is an inherited condition in which cholesterol levels are very high and atherosclerosis and heart attacks can, but do not always, occur very early in life. This condition is well recognized in the medical literature and can be diagnosed by special tests when total cholesterol, LDL cholesterol, and triglycerides are markedly elevated. Those unfortunate few who have inherited this condition have cholesterol levels over 350 mg/dl, sometimes as high as 1000. They lack what is known as LDL receptors on their cells. Thus, the LDL cholesterol is unable to enter their cells, and it builds up in the blood. However, their oxidized cholesterol does enter the cells of these people and con-tributes to a particular form of arterial disease that is pathologically distinct from the hardening of the arteries that affects the other 99% of the population. The important point is that the problems that these rare individuals experience cannot be extrapolated to the general population, 99% of whom do not have this inherited condition. For more on oxidized cholesterol, see chapter 4.

Chapter 2

Fat Chemistry-Simplified

In order to proceed with our understanding of the diet/cholesterol/heart disease question, I think it will be helpful to simplify the rather complex area of the chemistry of fats.

Fats (also called lipids) are organic substances that are not soluble in water. Fatty acids are chains of carbon atoms bonded together. At each bond are hydrogen atoms. The fat we eat and the fat in our bodies is in the form of triglycerides. Triglycerides consist of three fatty acid chains attached to a glycerol molecule.

The fatty acids are classified as **saturated** or **unsaturated**. The saturated fatty acids are relatively stable because the bonds between each carbon atom are filled with hydrogen atoms. Unsaturated fatty acids lack hydrogen atoms at specific bonding sites, which creates a **double** bond at that site. Double bonds are reactive and relatively unstable.

Monounsaturated fatty acids are lacking hydrogen atoms at one of the bonds. (They have one double bond.)

Polyunsaturated fatty acids have two or more double bond sites and are, thus, lacking four or more hydrogen atoms.

The polyunsaturated fatty acids are further classified into **Omega 3** or **Omega 6** fatty acids based on the location of the double bonds in the carbon chain. We will discuss the important distinction between omega 3 and omega 6 fats a little later.

Saturated fats are very stable and are solid at room temperature. They do not usually go rancid and they can be heated to the high temperatures involved in cooking without breaking down. The saturated fats in our food are generally found in food of animal origin and in coconut oil.

The monounsaturated fats, having only one double bond in each molecule, are also relatively stable. Hence, they can be stored at room temperature without becoming rancid and can be used in cooking, provided they are not heated to extremely high temperatures. The most common monounsaturated fatty acid in our food supply is oleic acid, which is the main component of olive oil. Monounsaturates are also found in avocados, almonds, pecans, peanuts, and cashews.

Polyunsaturated fatty acids, having more than one double bond in each molecule are relatively unstable. They can become rancid quickly. They are liquid even when refrigerated. Two of the polyunsaturated fatty acids are considered essential. The body cannot make them. They must be consumed in order to avoid essential fatty acid deficiency. The two essential fatty acids are alpha-linolenic acid (an omega 3), and linoleic acid, (an omega 6). **Polyunsaturated oils, such as corn oil, safflower oil, sunflower oil should never be used in cooking, because they will oxidize and break down into toxic substances.**

Actually, all fats in our food supply contain **combinations** of saturated, monounsaturated, and polyunsaturated fatty acids. Food of animal origin contains a relatively high proportion of saturated fatty acids. Olive oil contains mostly the monounsaturated oleic acid. The common vegetable oils such as corn oil, cottonseed oil, and sunflower oil, products grown in northern climates, contain mostly polyunsaturated fatty acids. The tropical oils, such as coconut and palm oil, on the other hand, contain mostly saturated fat and are solid at usual room temperature, but liquid in tropical climates.

Important to remember: Fats from **animal** origin are mostly **saturated**. (They do, however, also contain important unsaturated fats.)

Vegetable oils from northern climates are mostly **polyunsaturated**. Corn, safflower, sunflower, and cotton-seed oils are mostly Omega 6. Flax seed oil is a good vegetable source of Omega 3 fatty acids.

Olive oil is **monounsaturated.**

Coconut oil is mostly **saturated**.

Polyunsaturated oils (corn, safflower, cottonseed, soy oil) form up to 30% of modern diets. These oils consist of mostly omega 6 fatty acids. We have been told that they are good for us. The truth is that these oils, when consumed in excess (should be only about 4% of the diet) are known to contribute to cancer, heart disease, immune system problems, liver and lung damage, reproductive organ damage, digestive system problems, and impaired learning ability. The reason that these oils cause health problems is that they are readily oxidized to become toxic free radicals (see Chapter 4), particularly when exposed to heat and oxygen, as in cooking.

Cholesterol is a high molecular weight alcohol that is manufactured in our liver and in most human cells. It is also found in food from animal sources, such as meat, dairy products, butter, eggs. Cholesterol is a repair substance which plays many important roles in achieving and maintaining good health. In the next chapter we will discuss the many important functions of cholesterol and other fatty substances in the maintenance of good health.

Hydrogenated or partially hydrogenated oils are polyunsaturated oils (normally liquid at room temperature) which have been subjected to a chemical process which inserts hydrogen atoms into the unstable double bonds. This results in a stable, solid fat (shortening or margarine). This process begins with cheap rancid vegetable oils, which are subjected to high heat, metallic catalysts (usually nickel), bleaching, and more heat. Then emulsifiers and other additives are added. Then in the case of margarine, artificial coloring agents and flavors are added to make it resemble butter. Unfortunately, in the process of hydrogenation, the fatty acids are changed from the natural "cis" configuration to a toxic configuration called **"trans"**. The trans config-uration almost never occurs in nature. This subtle change in the shape of the fatty acid molecule causes profoundly devastating effects on the health of those who consume these unnatural fats.

Unfortunately, these partially hydrogenated oils (containing **trans** fats) are extremely prevalent in our food supply. They are found in virtually all commercial baked goods, breads, cookies, rolls, pastries, snack foods, chips, crackers, cereals, breakfast bars, candy bars, ice creams, even many so called "health food bars", fish sticks and other frozen foods such as frozen pot pies, packaged instant noodles, processed cheeses, even in baby foods, and of course in shortening such as Crisco, and margarines.

These partially hydrogenated oils (trans fats) are toxic to our bodies. They are absorbed from our digestive tract and assimilated into our cell membranes throughout the body. Our cell membranes, where all of our important life processes take place, are not able to function normally when these trans fats are integrated into the membrane. These altered fats block the uptake of essential fatty acids, which creates a cascade of devastation. Research has shown the following list of maladies to be associated with the intake of trans fats: Increased blood cholesterol, poor immune function, sexual dysfunction, cancer, atherosclerosis (hardening of the arteries), diabetes, obesity, birth defects, low-birth-weight babies, sterility, decreased visual acuity, difficulty with lactation. **Yes, these are the fats that have been promoted to the public for the last 50 years as being the healthy alternative. If you have been believing the advertising hype, as the majority of the American public have, you have been duped! Is it surprising that we have epidemics of heart disease, obesity, and diabetes?**

The food industry has been forced in recent years to acknowledge the dangers of the trans fats and has started to make margarines that are free of trans fats. My advice: trust mother nature. Butter is better! New laws are being passed to force food manufacturers to list trans fats on food labels. But this requirement will not be in effect until the year 2006.

Omega 3 Fats. These are the important fats for healthy metabolism, efficient fat burning, anti-inflammatory effects, brain power, normal brain and nervous system development in the developing fetus and the growing child. In our modern diets we are not consuming enough omega 3 fats, and we are consuming far too much of the omega 6 fats. There is a preponderance of omega 6 in the common polyunsaturated oils, such as corn oil, safflower oil, soy oil, and sunflower oil. So we are relatively deficient in omega 3 fats. The result of this imbalance, in addition to sluggish fat burning, is increased inflammation, increased tendency to form abnormal blood clots, high blood pressure, poor immune function, sterility, cancer, and weight gain. Best food sources for these important omega 3 fats are fish from northern oceans, such as salmon, cod, halibut, flax seed or its oil, wild game such as venison or pheasant, and grass-fed beef or buffalo.

Bottom line

- Avoid commercial unsaturated oils (corn oil, safflower oil, sunflower oil).

- Avoid trans fats (hydrogenated or partially hydrogenated oils). Always read labels on prepared processed foods, and avoid products containing these toxic fats.

- Consume flax seed, flax seed oil, cold water fish, fish oil supplements.

- Use flax seed oil or olive oil on salads and vegetables.

- Use butter in reasonable amounts.

- Best oil for coating pans in cooking is coconut oil. (It is stable, will not oxidize.)

Much of this information on fats, oils, and cholesterol is derived from the excellent website, www.westonaprice.org., with permission from Sally Fallon. Her book *Nourishing Traditions* is highly recommended.

Chapter 3

The Many Roles of Cholesterol and Saturated Fats

We have been warned by the medical profession, the pharmaceutical industry, the government, and the media to avoid saturated fats and cholesterol (animal fats). That by avoiding these fats and consuming the unsaturated and chemically altered fats such as margarine, we will be healthy and less likely to suffer heart attacks.

Is this good advice?

Let's take a look at the functions of saturated fats and cholesterol in the body.

First, the saturated fats.

- The saturated fatty acids make up more than 50% of our cell membranes. They give our cells necessary stiffness and integrity.

- They are the preferred food for the heart. <u>Yes, the main fuel for our heart's pumping action is saturated fat!</u> (Specifically, stearic acid and palmitic acid.) The fat around the heart that is used as a reserve of fuel is composed of saturated fat.

- They enhance our immune system.

- They are important for the health of our bones, by helping calcium to be incorporated into the bones.

- They are needed for utilization of essential fatty acids.

- They protect the liver from toxins, including alcohol. If you take Tylenol, a known liver toxin, saturated fat will help to protect your liver.

- Certain saturated fatty acids, the short and medium chain fatty acids, protect against infection.

NOW, WHAT ABOUT CHOLESTEROL?

- Cholesterol plays a role similar to saturated fat in our cell membranes. It helps to provide stiffness and stability. (Polyunsaturated fat provides fluidity to those same membranes. We need a balance of both.)

- Cholesterol is the precursor molecule for all of the important hormones in the body. This includes the corticosteroids, testosterone, estrogen, and progesterone.

- Cholesterol is the precursor for vitamin D. Exposure of our skin to sunshine converts cholesterol to vitamin D. This is the molecule that is so very important for bone formation and strength, for nervous system function, mineral metabolism, muscle tone, reproduction, insulin production, and immune function.

- Cholesterol acts as an antioxidant. As such it protects against free radical damage associated with toxins and advancing age. These free radical reactions are what lead to cancer and heart disease. This is a very important point. As we advance in age, our body naturally makes more cholesterol to protect us from the toxins and other insults that we are subjected to. Recent studies have noted an apparent protective role against infections for higher levels of blood cholesterol. These studies show that, among hospitalized patients, those who have low cholesterol have more infections.

- Cholesterol plays a role in the function of serotonin, the "feel good hormone". Low cholesterol levels (often the result of cholesterol lowering drugs) have been associated with depression, suicide, violent behavior, and aggression.

- Bile salts are made from cholesterol. Bile salts are important players in digestion and assimilation of fats.

- Cholesterol is present in abundance in breast milk. It plays an important role in the development of the brain and nervous system throughout the growing years.

- If we reduce the amount of cholesterol in our diet, our liver will compensate by making more.

Cholesterol is not the cause of heart disease! It is a potent antioxidant! A weapon against free radical toxins! And a repair substance that helps heal arterial damage!

High levels of cholesterol in the blood often indicate that the body needs extra protection from toxins. Among these toxins are the chemically altered fats. These are the fats that we have been told to consume, the trans fatty acids that are found in margarine and almost all commercial breads, baked goods, processed snacks, crackers, cookies, salad dressing, whipped topping, many candies, most ice creams, and many other processed foods.

When the body is detoxified through a healthy diet and lifestyle, and when it is protected from toxins by appropriate consumption of antioxidant nutrients, the need for protection from toxins is decreased, and cholesterol levels decrease naturally.

No, the advice to avoid the saturated fats and cholesterol found in meat, dairy products, and eggs is not good advice! We need these fats in <u>moderate</u> amounts as part of a well-planned diet that includes vegetables, fruits and naturally occurring omega 3 fats and monounsaturated fats. These are healthy fats! On the other hand, the trans fats found in partially hydrogenated oils, margarines, and shortenings are one of the significant causes of atherosclerosis, heart attacks, cancer, and many of the other degenerative diseases. Those are the fats to avoid!

Chapter 4

Free Radicals, Oxidized Cholesterol, Antioxidants

Oxygen is stable when it occurs as two molecules together (O2). When we are exposed to toxins such as smog, chemicals, chlorine in drinking water, toxic metals, **trans fats**, and even in the normal process of burning food for energy, this O2 molecule is split, resulting in an unstable oxygen radical, a "free radical". This free radical, which lacks an electron, steals electrons from other molecules, causing damage to tissues throughout the body. This free radical activity is at the very basis of most disease, particularly the degenerative diseases associated with aging. It results in inflammation, cancer, high blood pressure, cataracts, heart disease, Alzheimer's disease, and arthritis. It is one of the major causes of premature aging, wrinkled skin, and age spots. Yes, free radicals are involved in the development of almost every known ailment.

Fortunately we have marvelous defense systems to fight off free radical damage. Antioxidants are nutrients that protect us against the damage that free radicals cause. The most well known antioxidants are vitamin C, and vitamin E. A few of the many others are vitamin A, vitamin B2, magnesium, zinc, selenium, co-enzyme Q-10, glutamine, taurine, and lipoic acid. And, yes, cholesterol itself is a potent antioxidant that protects and repairs the walls of our arteries when they are damaged by toxins like trans fats, cigarette smoke, and toxic metals like lead, mercury, and cadmium.

But cholesterol itself can become oxidized to form oxycholesterol. Cholesterol becomes oxidized by free radical activity. The oxidized form of cholesterol is believed to be a cause of arterial inflammation, which results in high blood pressure and heart attacks. So you can see that the problem is not the level of cholesterol in your blood, but the free radical activity that is oxidizing your cholesterol into a toxic molecule. And what is one of the major toxins oxidizing your cholesterol? **Trans fats!** Yes, those toxic fats present in margarine, shortening, commercial baked goods, crackers, cookies, salad dressings, even some ice creams, and numerous other prepared and packaged foods. **Always read labels!**

What about french fries and other fried foods? Heating unsaturated oils like safflower, soy, corn, or cottonseed oil to the high temperatures used in frying causes oxidation of these unstable fatty acids resulting in the generation of massive amounts of toxic free radicals. When these oils are repeatedly heated, as they usually are in restaurants and donut shops, the toxicity increases with each reheating. **Important message:** Avoid french fries, donuts, potato chips, deep fried chicken and fish, and all foods fried at high temperature.

If you fry food at home, the safest oil to use is coconut oil. It is available in health food stores. Reason: It is highly saturated. (No double bonds to react with oxygen to create free radicals.) Next best choice is old-fashioned lard. In any case, do not heat oils excessively, as it is the high heat which causes toxic breakdown and free radical generation.

Chapter 5

Good Cholesterol-Bad Cholesterol. What's it all about?

Cholesterol, being insoluble in water and in blood, is carried around in the blood surrounded by spheres of fat and protein called lipoproteins, kind of like little submarines. The outer layer of these spheres is a water-soluble protein which can carry the cholesterol through cell membranes into our cells.

These lipoproteins are named according to their density. HDL is high density lipoprotein, and LDL is low density lipoprotein. HDL is the so-called "good cholesterol", and LDL is the so-called "bad cholesterol". The HDL carries cholesterol from artery walls and other tissues to the liver where the cholesterol can be made into important hormones or excreted in the bile. The LDL carries cholesterol from the liver to the peripheral tissues including the arterial walls. When cells need cholesterol, the LDL submarines deliver it to the interior of the cells. Most of the cholesterol in the blood is carried by the LDL, and a smaller amount is carried by the HDL.

Uffe Ravnskov, M.D., author of the extremely well researched and documented book, *The Cholesterol Myths* poses the question, *Why is a natural substance with important biological functions called "bad" when it is transported from the liver to the peripheral tissues by LDL, and "good" when it is transported the other way by HDL?* The reason is that a number of studies have shown that relatively low HDL and high LDL are associated with a greater risk of heart attack, and high HDL and low LDL are associated with lesser risk. Stated another way, a low HDL/LDL ratio is a "risk factor" for heart disease. However, Ravnskov points out the very important fact that a risk factor is not necessarily a cause. In his brilliant analysis of the many studies on the diet/cholesterol/heart connection he brings out the point that factors such as smoking, sedentary lifestyle, obesity, and stress will cause a low HDL/LDL ratio, and will also cause heart attacks. The very important point is that a low HDL/LDL ratio is a reflection of these other factors, and not a cause of the heart attacks. In the same manner, elevated total cholesterol is sometimes associated with heart attacks, and is thus called a risk factor. **But, again, a risk factor is not the same as a cause.**

Chapter 6

Statin Drugs
The Multi-Billion Dollar Experiment

You've seen the ads. Lipitor! Zocor! Pravichol! Crestor! Smiling happy people pleased that their cholesterol numbers have dropped!

Most doctors have been convinced by the pharmaceutical industry, through their multi-million dollar advertising campaigns, and through the pharmaceutical company representatives who visit their offices, that studies show that patients taking these drugs have an improved chance of avoiding a heart attack, and of avoiding heart attack death. And, indeed, some of the studies do show that.

But there are some serious problems with the studies. A few of the problems:

- The statins are effective in lowering risk of heart attack in groups of individuals for whom cholesterol is not considered a risk factor, such as women, and elderly individuals. **All studies have shown that cholesterol is either a weak risk factor or not a risk factor at all in women, and in men over 50.**

- The statins protected against heart attacks whether the individual's cholesterol was high or low.

- There was no association between the degree of cholesterol lowering and the outcome.

If the statins protect against heart attacks in groups of people for whom cholesterol is not a risk factor, and if they protect, whether cholesterol is high or low, and if the amount of cholesterol reduction is not a factor, then it would appear that something other than cholesterol lowering is going on with the statins. Perhaps the statins do more than lower cholesterol. Yes, that is exactly the case! It has been shown that by inhibiting a substance called mevalonate, not only is cholesterol production inhibited, but certain other factors involved in development of atherosclerosis are inhibited as well. Specifically, platelet aggregation (stickiness) and adhesion molecule activity are inhibited. These are good things, because these are important steps in the progression of arterial disease and abnormal clotting. It is also believed that the statins inhibit the inflammation that is part of the atherosclerotic process.

Yes, the statins do give some protection against heart attacks, but it is not due to cholesterol reduction. As Dr. Ravnskov puts it, *The proponents of the cholesterol hypothesis have simply had incredible luck in finding a substance that prevents cardiovascular disease, and at the same time, lowers cholesterol.*

How much benefit, how much risk reduction is actually demonstrated in the studies that are being used to promote this multi-billion dollar human experiment? Here, again, we see that by cleverly focusing on certain statistical numbers to the exclusion of other equally important or perhaps more important numbers, the perception of benefit is greatly exaggerated. Looking at "relative risk reduction" and ignoring "absolute risk reduction" (statistical terms poorly understood by most people, including practicing physicians), gives the impression that the risk of dying from a heart attack is reduced in a major way, when actually the risk reduction in absolute terms in all of the studies was minimal. For example, in the Scandinavian Simvastatin Survival Study, a patient with pre-existing artery disease, the chance of not dying from a heart attack over a 4 to 6 year period was about 92%. With statin treatment it was about 95%, a 3% difference. For a healthy person who does not have pre-existing heart and artery disease, the results are even less impressive. The healthy person in the WOSCOPS (West of Scotland Coronary Prevention Study) had a 98.4% chance of not dying of heart disease without treatment, versus a 98.8% chance of not dying with statin treatment. A 0.4% difference. There are many such examples detailed by Dr. Ravnskov in *The Cholesterol Myths*. Most of the studies that have shown decreased deaths from heart attacks have also shown an increase in deaths from other causes.

Benefit to Risk Ratio. This is a concept used by the healing professions to determine if a particular treatment is appropriate for a particular condition. We have discussed the benefits of statin treatment and found them to be minimal. What do we know about the risks and costs?

At a very significant dollar cost per year, a person taking any of the statin drugs is at risk for a very formidable list of side effects and adverse reactions. Just a small portion of this list includes hepatitis, pancreatitis, jaundice, muscle cramps, muscle pain, rhabdomyolysis (a severe and sometimes fatal painful muscle deterioration), tremor, dizziness, anxiety, insomnia, depression, hair loss, itching skin, gynecomastia (breast swelling in men), loss of libido, erectile dysfunction. These reactions and more are listed in the Physicians Desk Reference (PDR).

A very alarming side effect of the statin drugs has recently come to the attention of those who have an interest in such matters through the publication of *Lipitor, Thief of Memory—Statin Drugs and the Misguided War on Cholesterol* by physician and ex-astronaut, Duane Graveline, M.D. In this extremely well written and expertly documented book, he talks of his harrowing personal experience with "transient global amnesia" which occurred as a result of his taking the statin drug, Lipitor. This is a very alarming condition where, for several hours, the person so afflicted is totally unable to form new memory. Even very important events, which have happened only moments before, are completely absent from his memory. Sometimes the return of memory function is incomplete. This condition and other mental function problems, such as forgetfulness and loss of ability to concentrate, are occurring with increasing frequency as the statin drugs are prescribed to increasing numbers of people. Since most doctors and patients are unaware that these brain malfunctions can be a side effect of statin drugs, the conditions are usually misdiagnosed as senility, mini-strokes, or early Alzheimer's disease. In Dr. Graveline's fascinating book he is attempting to bring these alarming and potentially imperiling side effects of statin drugs to the attention of the general public, and particularly to the attention of the medical profession and the manufacturers of the statin drugs.

Another serious problem associated with all of the statin drugs, which is well known to the manufacturers, but is not listed in the PDR or on package inserts and thus is unknown to most physicians, is that by suppressing the enzyme responsible for manufacturing cholesterol in the liver (known as HMG CoA Reductase), the drugs also suppress the liver's production of CoEnzyme Q10 (CoQ10). This is a substance which plays an extremely important role in energy production in the heart muscle and in every cell in the body. CoQ10 is manufactured primarily in the liver, is found only in trace amounts in food, and is available as a supplement. Its reduction by statin drugs in a relatively healthy young person is not likely to have noticeable adverse consequences, but in a person with existing heart disease or in a feeble elderly person, it can lead to decreased efficiency of heart muscle contractions, which can eventually result in congestive heart failure. **Yes, the highly acclaimed statin drugs, aggressively promoted to reduce the risk of heart disease can be a causative factor in the development of**

congestive heart failure. In recent years there has been a significant increase in the incidence of congestive heart failure, and the widespread use of the statin drugs is suspected of being the major cause.

In the words of researcher and practicing cardiologist, Peter H. Langsjoen, M.D., *In my practice of 19 years in Tyler, Texas, I have seen a frightening increase in heart failure secondary to statin usage, "statin cardiomyopathy". Over the past five years, statins have become more potent, are being prescribed in higher doses, and are being used with reckless abandon in the elderly and in patients with "normal" cholesterol levels. We are in the midst of a congestive heart failure epidemic in the US with a dramatic increase over the past decade. Are we contributing to this epidemic through our zealous use of statins? In large part I think the answer is yes. We are now in a position to witness the unfolding of the greatest medical tragedy of all time. Never before in history has the medical establishment knowingly (Merck & Co., Inc. has two 1990 patents combining CoQ10 with statins to prevent CoQ10 depletion and attendant side effects) created a life threatening nutrient deficiency in millions of otherwise healthy people, only to sit back with arrogance and horrific irresponsibility and watch to see what happens. As I see two to three new statin cardiomyopathies per week in my practice, I cannot help but view my once great profession with a mixture of sorrow and contempt.*

This dangerous suppression of CoQ10 production by statin drugs warrants a warning in the advertisements for statin drugs in Canada, but curiously, no such warning occurs in the United States statin drug ads.

Another warning that occurs in the Canadian ads for statins that is noticeably absent from the U.S ads is: *the beneficial effects of lowering LDL cholesterol may be blunted by a concomitant increase in Lp(a).* We know from the early

36

work of Linus Pauling, Ph.D. and Matthias Rath, M.D., and now many others, that elevated Lp(a) is considered to be a more important risk factor for predicting heart disease than LDL cholesterol. See chapter 17.

One more very important point regarding statin drugs, which also applies to some of the earlier cholesterol lowering drugs as well. In studies utilizing rodents, all of these drugs produced cancer. What about possible cancer causation in humans? It generally takes many years for cancer to develop from exposure to a cancer causing substance, and these drugs have not been around long enough for that to happen. But in the CARE (Cholesterol and Recurrent Events) trial, there was a very significant incidence of breast cancer in those who took Pravachol (a statin drug), compared to those in the control group. The ultimate effects of treating millions of people with these drugs will not be known for many years.

Let's not fail to factor in the significant cost and incon-venience of the periodic office visits to the doctor for lab tests to monitor levels of cholesterol and other lipids and to check for damage to the liver and/or the muscles.

For an excellent review article on the risk/benefit ratio of taking statin drugs, I recommend *Statin Drugs--A Critical Review of the Risk/Benefit Clinical Research* by Joel Kauffman, Ph.D. It can be found at www.drugintel.com.

Bottom line: For a very significant cost in dollars, and at a significant risk of side effects and adverse reactions, including the risk of death, the statin drugs may provide a small reduction in risk of heart attacks. However, the benefit is not related to lowering of cholesterol, but to reducing other factors which are involved in the development of heart and artery disease.

For better, cheaper, safer, more natural methods of achieving reduction of the factors that lead to heart attacks, read on!

Chapter 7

Summary of What We Know at This Point

- Eating animal fat and cholesterol do not significantly raise blood cholesterol levels.

- Cholesterol plays many important roles in our bodies. Our bodies produce 3 to 4 times more cholesterol than we eat.

- People with low cholesterol are just as likely to die of heart disease as those with high cholesterol.

- People with low cholesterol are more likely to die of stroke, cancer, suicide, and accidents, particularly when cholesterol has been lowered by drugs.

- Statin drugs can reduce slightly the risk of having a heart attack and of dying of a heart attack, but at significant cost in dollars, side effects, and possible serious adverse reactions, including death.

- Evidence exists that the benefit of statins is due not to lowering of cholesterol, but to other mechanisms.

Now that we have established the lack of importance of lowering cholesterol, now that we can stop worrying about our cholesterol levels, we will address the more important questions of: **What are the real causes of heart disease, and how do we prevent and successfully reverse it?** We'll get to that and also discuss the current epidemics of obesity and diabetes in Part II of this book.

But first, let's take a look at what some renowned scientific researchers who disagree with the mainstream diet/ cholesterol/heart disease concepts have to say.

Chapter 8

Voices of Dissent

You have been led to believe that all responsible scientists support the diet/cholesterol/heart disease connection. The truth is that there has been a great deal of dissent among the scientific community. Many responsible scientists have strongly criticized the diet/cholesterol/heart disease connection. However, their dissent has only been published in journals and books that are not widely accessible to the general public. And their voices have been drowned out by the powerful voices of the medical/pharmaceutical/food industry establishment that has much to gain by the ever expanding use of vegetable oils and other synthetic foods, and the ever expanding prescription of cholesterol reducing drugs.

I will cite just a few examples.

George Mann, M.D., a now retired professor of medicine and biochemistry at Vanderbilt University, has called the diet/cholesterol/heart idea the *greatest scientific deception of our time.* Regarding the cholesterol lowering trials, he says, *Never in the history of science have so many costly experiments failed so consistently.* About the Lipid Research Clinics trial he writes that the unsupportive results have not prevented its directors from *bragging about this cataclysmic breakthrough.* He further states, *Fearing to lose their soft money funding, the academicians who should speak up and stop this wasteful anti-science are strangely* *quiet. Their silence has delayed a solution for coronary heart disease by a generation.*

In 1973 **Edward Pinckney, M.D.**, an editor of four medical journals and former co-editor of the prestigious Journal of the American Medical Association, published *The Cholesterol Controversy*, a book which summarized the inconsistencies in the diet/cholesterol/heart idea. In the beginning of his book he states, *Your fear of dying, if you happen to be one of the great many people who suffer from this morbid preoccupation, may well have made you a victim of the cholesterol controversy. For if you have come to believe that you can ward off death from heart disease by altering the amount of cholesterol in your blood, whether by diet or drugs, you are following a regimen that has no basis in fact. Rather, you, as a consumer, have been taken in by certain commercial interests and health groups who are more interested in your money than your life.* Those thoughts, so well expressed in 1973, are perhaps even more valid today, as the cholesterol experiment has become a multi-billion dollar industry.

Paul J. Rosch, M.D., president of the American Institute of Stress, and clinical professor of medicine and psychiatry at New York Medical College, is editor of three medical journals. He has been president of the New York State Society of Internal Medicine, and has written extensively on the role of stress in heart disease and cancer. He has appeared on many popular TV shows, been interviewed and quoted in many major newspapers and magazines, and has published several articles regarding the cholesterol hypothesis and diet/cholesterol/heart concepts. Dr. Rosch concludes *A massive crusade has been conceived to lower your cholesterol count by rigidly restricting dietary fat, coupled with aggressive drug treatment. Much of the impetus for this comes from speculation, rather than any solid scientific proof.* He continues, *The public is so brainwashed that many people believe that the lower your* *cholesterol, the healthier you will be, or the longer you will live. Nothing could be further from the truth.* To explain how this conspiracy could be pulled off and maintained for so many years, he states, *The cholesterol cartel of drug companies, manufacturers of low-fat foods, blood-testing devices, and others with huge vested financial interests have waged a highly successful promotional campaign. Their power is so great that they have infiltrated medical and government regulatory agencies that would normally protect us from such dogma.*

Ray Rosenman, M.D. is the retired Director of Cardiovascular Research in the Health Sciences Program at SRI International in Menlo Park, California. Also Chief of Medicine at Mount Zion Hospital and Medical Center in San Francisco, an author of four books and many articles and textbook chapters on cardiovascular disease, he has written several reviews of the diet/cholesterol/heart connection. Here is the conclusion from his most recent review. *These data lead to a conclusion that neither diet, serum lipids, nor their changes can explain wide national and regional differences of ischemic heart disease (coronary heart disease) rates, nor the variable 20th century rises and declines of CHD mortality.*

This conclusion is supported by the results of many clinical trials which fail to provide adequate evidence that lowering serum cholesterol, particularly by dietary changes, is associated with a significant reduction of CHD mortality or improved longevity. It is variously stated that the preventive effects of dietary and drug treatments have been exaggerated by a tendency in trial reports, reviews, and other papers to cite and inflate supportive results, while suppressing discordant data, and many such examples are cited.

Russell Smith, M.D., working along with Dr. Pinkney produced two large thoroughly documented and referenced volumes on the diet/cholesterol/heart disease subject. Regarding the quality of research used to promote the cholesterol conspiracy, he stated, *...much of the epidemiologic research is, in fact, rather imprecise and understandably so, because it has been conducted principally by individuals with no formal education and little on-the-job training in the scientific method. Consequently, studies are often poorly designed and data are often inappropriately analyzed and interpreted. Moreover, biases are so commonplace, they appear to be the rule, rather than the exception. It is virtually impossible not to recognize that many researchers routinely manipulate and/or interpret their data to fit preconceived hypotheses, rather than manipulate hypotheses to fit their data. Much of the literature, therefore, is nothing less than an affront to the discipline of science.*

The current campaign to convince every American to change his or her diet and, in many cases to initiate drug 'therapy' for life is based on fabrications, erroneous interpretations and /or gross exaggerations of findings and, very importantly, the ignoring of massive amounts of unsupportive data....It does not seem possible that objective scientists without vested interests could ever interpret the literature as supportive.

Recognizing the power of the institutions behind the cholesterol conspiracy, and calling their work *incompetent and sloppy* he states, *The political and financial power of the National Heart Lung and Blood Institute and the American Heart Association team...is enormous and without equal. And because the alliance has substantial credibility in the eyes of the public and most practicing physicians, it has become a juggernaut, able to use its power and prestige to suppress a great body of unsupportive evidence and even defy the most fundamental tool of scientists, logic.*

William E. Stehbens, M.D., Professor in the Department of Pathology at Wellington School of Medicine in New Zealand has reviewed the diet/cholesterol/heart questions in several thorough articles. Among his many critical comments regarding the quality of the science used by the supporters of the cholesterol myth is this *...It is essential to adhere to hard scientific facts and logic. Scientific evidence for the role of dietary fat and hypercholesterolemia in the causation of atherosclerosis is seriously lacking. ...The lipid hypothesis has enjoyed undeserved longevity and respectability. Readers should be aware of the unscientific nature of claims used to support it and see it as little more than a pernicious bum steer.*

These brief quotes are just a small sampling of the volumes of dissent that have been published. Chapter 9 in Dr. Ravnskov's *The Cholesterol Myths* quotes these and several others, complete with references, which will allow the serious reader to find and read the original papers in order to have a more complete appreciation of the massive quantity of research that contradicts the diet/cholesterol/heart disease connection.

Part II

What Really Matters?

Man will occasionally stumble over the truth, but usually manages to pick himself up, walk over or around it, and carry on. **Winston S. Churchill**

If cholesterol is not really important in predicting heart disease; if avoiding cholesterol and animal fats is not helpful and could even be harmful; if lowering cholesterol by diet and drugs can cause more problems than it can prevent, then what are the real causes of our epidemic of heart disease? And, more important, what can we do to prevent heart attacks, stop the progress of arterial disease, and even reverse it? What can we do in this modern toxic world we live in to maximize our chances of leading a long healthy life?

What are the real causes of heart disease? Actually there are several causes, most of which we can do something about. The one factor that we cannot change is our genetic inheritance. Some of us have inherited genetic tendencies, which will predispose us toward heart disease. But even in that situation, we can alter our destiny, avoid heart disease, reverse it if it is present, and increase our health and lifespan. We can enjoy our golden years in good health.

We have established that LDL cholesterol is an unreliable predictor of heart disease risk, but not a cause of heart disease. So now we will focus on some of the real causes of heart disease, causes based on solid scientific evidence. Fortunately, these factors can be dealt with by relatively easy and inexpensive changes in our diet and lifestyle, and by taking a few scientifically researched nutritional supplements. For those already dealing with significant heart and blood vessel disease, there are natural alternative treatments available through skilled, well-qualified physicians to reverse even advanced illness.

Chapter 9

The Homocysteine Story

Homocysteine: an amino acid that under certain circumstances accumulates to toxic levels and plays a key role in the causation of cardiovascular disease, Alzheimer's disease, and other chronic degenerative diseases.

In 1969 Kilmer S. McCully, M.D., a graduate of Harvard Medical School published the first article relating homocysteine to atherosclerosis. His continuing research eventually established that an elevated level of homocysteine in the blood was a very important cause, probably the most important cause of atherosclerotic heart disease. He was, at the time, a scientist doing research at the prestigious Massachusetts General Hospital. This first article was followed by much research and more articles by McCully, and eventually by many other researchers throughout the world.

Not surprisingly, McCully's ideas on an alternative explanation for the cause of heart disease in the early 1970s were not welcomed by the medical/pharmaceutical establishment. The cholesterol bandwagon was beginning to roll. Many people, the big institutions, and the pharmaceutical companies were heavily invested. Science be damned! They wanted no interference with the huge profits to be made from the cholesterol campaign.

As a result of his efforts to enlighten his colleagues and the rest of the scientific community, McCully lost his research grants and became a *persona non grata* to the medical research community. He was blackballed by the Massachusetts General Hospital and Harvard Medical School power structures, and for many years was unable to get a research position anywhere in the country. After a long and expensive effort, eventually involving legal action against Massachusetts General Hospital and Harvard Medical School, he was hired to continue his research at the VA Hospital in Providence, Rhode Island. Since 2001 he has continued his research at the VA Hospital in Boston, Massachusetts, where he functions also as chief of pathology.

By the 1990s several researchers in various European countries began to confirm McCully's ideas about the role of elevated homocysteine levels in causing heart disease. Finally, in the late 1990s, the homocysteine story began to receive some of the recognition that it deserved. Articles on the correlation between homocysteine and heart disease appeared in the New England Journal of Medicine, and the Journal of the American Medical Association. Shortly thereafter, stories about this newly discovered cause of heart disease appeared in Time and Newsweek magazines and also in The Saturday Evening Post. There is now such a high level of interest in homocysteine, that, according to a recent conversation with Dr. McCully, research articles on the subject are being published at the rate of 3 to 4 per day. In recent years the medical profession has begun to catch on, but even now, all too often a medical screening for heart disease risk looks only at cholesterol, HDL, LDL, and triglycerides. Or sometimes, just total cholesterol. As we will see, a test for homocysteine is a far more important measurement.

In simplest terms, when homocysteine is elevated, it causes damage to the lining of arterial walls, which leads to heart disease.   Adequate amounts of certain vitamins (vitamin B12, vitamin B6, and folic acid) reduce homocysteine to normal levels and prevent arterial damage and heart disease.

To quote Kilmer McCully, who has been called "The Father of Homocysteine" from his excellent book, *The Heart Revolution*. *The message of this 'heart revolution' is simple and clear. Heart disease is caused by modern processed food, and the way to prevent the disease is to improve the quality of your diet. Heart disease is a modern disease because it is manmade. If we ate what our bodies needed, heart disease would be as rare as it is in unindustrialized parts of the world. That would be a revolution.*

Homocysteine is an amino acid that is created from the essential amino acid, methionine. Red meats, chicken, fish, garlic, onions, and beans are among the foods that are high in methionine. We need methionine, but under certain circumstances, the conversion of methionine to homocysteine becomes excessive, and homocysteine builds up to toxic levels and causes the damage to arterial walls that leads to heart disease. Adequate levels of folic acid, vitamin B12, and vitamin B6 will generally keep active the detoxification pathways that prevent homocysteine from rising to toxic levels.   The deterioration of the modern diet, with the excessive consumption of processed devitalized foods, and the absence of nutritious whole foods has resulted in widespread nutritional deficiencies of these important vitamins that would otherwise keep homocysteine at safe non-toxic levels.

Yes, atherosclerotic heart disease is, to a large extent, a nutritional deficiency disease. It is not caused by too much fat and cholesterol, but by the absence of the important nutrients that prevent the accumulation of toxic levels of homocysteine. We are not consuming enough of the important foods that contain the vitamins required to keep homocysteine at a safe low level.

As knowledge regarding homocysteine continues to expand, scientists are now realizing that elevated levels of homocysteine play a role not only in heart disease, but also in many of the other chronic diseases associated with aging.

How does that happen?

An important basic process called methylation is essential to DNA repair, the process by which our worn out tissues are rebuilt. Elevated homocysteine can be a sign of defective methylation. The resulting defective DNA repair results in accelerated aging. Elevated homocysteine indicates that the methylation cycle is malfunctioning. Efficient methylation is essential for normal healthy aging. Defective methylation is productive of accelerated aging, heart disease, and even the dreaded Alzheimer's disease.

Studies have shown that among the elderly who do not take vitamin supplements, nutrient deficiencies are extremely common, particularly deficiencies of vitamin B12, folic acid, and vitamin B6, the B vitamins that are important to prevent heart disease, Alzheimer's disease, and many of the other diseases and discomforts of aging.

A gradually increasing memory loss and personality change may signal the onset of Alzheimer's disease, or it may simply be the result of vitamin deficiencies. These deficiencies can produce memory failure, depression, and mood disorders in the absence of Alzheimer's disease. In any case, it makes good sense to get a homocysteine blood test and to supplement with a good vitamin B complex supplement, or a high quality multi-vitamin that contains adequate levels of B12, folic acid, and B6 whether homocysteine is elevated or not. More specific recommendations will be discussed a little later.

Will simply taking these B vitamins be enough to avoid a heart attack?

Taking these vitamins is a very important first step. The usual recommended doses will be enough to normalize homocysteine levels in most people. However, some folks will require higher than usual doses because of particular inherited enzyme deficiencies and/or toxic lifestyle factors such as smoking, obesity, or exposure to toxic environmental factors. Levels of homocysteine in your blood can help determine if your doses are adequate.

What is a healthy homocysteine level. Actually, the lower the level, the less risk for heart attack. The usual normal range is given as 5 to 10 micromoles per liter. However, the journal "Circulation" in 1995 published the following ranges and risk indications.

- 0 – 6.3   Lowest risk
- 6.3 – 10   Moderate risk
- Over 10   Highest risk

So if your reading is over 7, you've got some work to do, some changes to make.

While these three B vitamins are a very important part of reducing heart disease risk, they are just a small part of what is lacking in the typical modern diets in our so-called civilized world. Yes, taking these three vitamins in adequate amounts will lower your homocysteine to safe levels, and thereby go a long way toward preventing heart disease. But there is more to aging healthfully, gracefully, and vigorously than simply avoiding a heart attack.

Our modern diets are much too high in refined carbohydrates (white flour products, sugar, white rice, pastas) and other highly refined processed devitalized foods. These are the foods that contribute to premature aging and chronic degenerative disease. For vigorous health we must return to the diets of our ancestors and include physical exercise in our daily lives. More on that in later chapters.

What are adequate levels of these important B vitamins? It depends on whom you read.

Here are the amounts recommended by Dr. McCully, depending on adequacy of food intake and current health condition.

- Low risk person with homocysteine below 8 and following Mc Cully's "Health Revolution" diet.

  No supplements.

- Mild risk. Homocysteine between 8 and 12.

Daily dose:	Folic acid	400 mcg.
	B12	100 mcg.
	B6	3 mg.

- High risk. Homocysteine between 12 and 20 and/or family history of heart disease, obesity, smoker, high blood pressure, high LDL, low HDL.

Daily dose:	Folic acid	2000 mcg.
	B12	500 mcg.
	B6	50 mg.

- Very high risk. Homocysteine between 16 and 30 and/or angina, ischemic attacks, kidney failure, diabetes.

Daily dose:	Folic acid	5000 mcg.
	B12	1000 mcg.
	B6	100 mg.

There are many other nutrients that are helpful to prevent and treat heart disease and favor healthy aging.

Considerably more nutritional help and medical attention is needed for the person with significant risk factors and for the person with established heart disease.

Many health practitioners, who are aware of the important role that nutrients play in health and disease, are recommending higher levels of these important B vitamins for heart disease prevention, and also advising that the upper limit of a safe homocysteine level be placed at 6.3. In simple terms, the lower the homocysteine, the better! Other important nutrients for healthy heart function will be discussed in a later chapter.

Obviously, the person at high risk should utilize a more aggressive regimen than one who is young, in good health, and following a healthy diet. If you are at high risk or already have a heart related illness, it is very important that you seek competent medical help. You will find a list of resources for finding nutritionally trained physicians and other health care practitioners in the appendix of this book.

Is there a relationship between LDL "bad" cholesterol and homocysteine? Based on Kilmer McCully's research, the LDL cholesterol transports the toxic homocysteine molecules to the arterial wall where they do their damage. If homocysteine is kept at minimal levels through adequate vitamin intake, and a healthy diet and lifestyle, there is far less concern over elevated LDL. If there is an advantage to be gained by lowering our LDL, it is that there will be less homocysteine delivered to the arterial wall.

One more point! We've discussed oxycholesterol (cholesterol containing extra oxygen atoms). This is the form of cholesterol that can cause arterial damage. The cholesterol that occurs in eggs, meats, and dairy products, in its natural state, does not cause arterial damage, but oxidized cholesterol can. Oxycholesterol occurs when the cholesterol in foods is over-heated, or processed. These oxycholesterols are present in powdered eggs, powdered milk, fried meats. But there is another source of these dangerous oxycholesterols <u>within</u> the body. Homocysteine can cause oxidation of cholesterol within the cells of the body to form oxycholesterols. So we must try to avoid the foods containing the oxidized cholesterol, but we must also try to prevent the oxidation of the cholesterol within the cells of our body by keeping our homocysteine low.

Sound a little complicated? Perhaps it is, but the solution is actually rather simple. Eat your vegetables, fruits, fresh lean meats, eggs, and whole grains. Avoid processed foods, synthetic, factory-made fake foods and foods fried at high temperature.

To summarize: The cause of our epidemic of heart disease is the change from the healthy diets of our ancestors to the present nutritionally deficient over-processed, toxin-laden diets that the vast majority of modern civilization attempts to survive on. The solution becomes obvious. Return to the healthy foods that nourished our ancestors, and supplement with the important nutrients that we've been missing.

Chapter 10

Screening Tests for Heart Disease

Beyond Homocysteine

Realizing that the usual lipid profiles actually have little value in assessing heart disease risk, there are now several valuable laboratory tests, in addition to the very important homocysteine level, that are increasingly being utilized by astute physicians to more accurately predict the likelihood of heart disease. These are used, of course, in addition to a complete detailed medical history, thorough physical examination, and appropriate non-invasive testing pro-cedures.

Here are some of the lab tests that are definitely worth pursuing. This is not meant to be a complete list. The experienced, well-educated, up-to-date physician will have other laboratory tests that he/she feels are equally important.

Lipoprotein(a). Referred to as Lp(a) (or LP little a), lipoprotein(a) is believed to be the lipid that begins the process that results in the formation of atherosclerotic plaque. I believe it is not only a risk factor, but unlike cholesterol, when it is elevated it actually plays a role in causation of arterial disease. Lp(a) is believed to be an artery repair substance. It is involved in the laying down of plaque over injured areas of arteries. But when this process overshoots, the plaque buildup begins to impair blood flow.

For more on dealing with elevated levels of LP(a), see chapter 17 on the Linus Pauling-Matthias Rath treatment for preventing and reversing heart disease.

C-Reactive Protein-HS. (CRP) It is now being recognized that chronic inflammation is a major factor in the development and progression of arterial disease. C-Reactive Protein is a test that measures a protein that increases in the presence of inflammation. The HS simply stands for "high sensitivity". If CRP is significantly elevated in the absence of an obvious infection (such as a cold, bronchitis, urinary tract infection, abscess, pneumonia, etc.) or an injury, this is considered to represent a high risk for heart attack. Often a chronic low-grade infection, such as a gum or tooth infection, is contributing to this inflammatory state. These infections, if present, should be adequately treated to minimize heart disease risk. At this time researchers are not clear as to whether the C-Reactive Protein is just a marker for inflammation, or if it actually plays a causative role in arterial inflammation. Since the discovery of the relationship between elevated CRP and heart disease is relatively recent, there is no general agreement as to the appropriate treatment for the inflammation signaled by elevated CRP. Niacin has been used successfully for treatment, as have the statin drugs (at the risk of developing the serious side effects previously discussed). A holistic, low-stress life style, a healthy diet, and avoidance of smoking and other toxic exposures will help deal with elevated CRP at the same time that it is lowering homocysteine levels. Certain nutritional supplements can help to reduce the inflammation signaled by elevated CRP. See chapter 13 for supplement recommendations.

Fibrinogen is a protein in the blood that plays a role in normal clotting following an injury, such as a laceration. If it is elevated in the absence of injury it can increase the likelihood of abnormal clots and heart attacks. Smoking, obesity, and the other factors that increase CRP also tend to increase fibrinogen. Weight normalization, smoking cessation, healthful whole food nutrition, and exercise tend to reduce fibrinogen levels toward normal.

Insulin is a hormone released by the pancreas that helps to control the level of sugar in your blood by helping the sugar enter your cells where it is needed for energy. It is important to know that insulin is also responsible for storing excess sugar in the form of fat. Since sugar and other carbohydrates play an important role in obesity, diabetes, and heart disease, it is important to define some terms. Carbohydrates are foods that are loaded with sugars or complexes of sugars. Simple carbohydrates contain sugars that are easily and rapidly digested. Complex carbohydrates contain sugars arranged in long complexes, which are slowly digested. The simple sugars are rapidly absorbed causing increases in blood sugar levels. White sugar, high fructose corn syrup, white flour, white rice, honey, maple syrup, fruit and fruit juices are examples of simple sugars. Foods such as whole grains, corn, lentils, beans, leafy green vegetables, and potatoes are complex carbohydrates. The more sugar and other carbohydrates one eats, the more insulin is released by the pancreas, resulting in progressively higher blood insulin levels. Gradually the cells of the body become increasingly resistant to normal levels of insulin, so that the pancreas must secrete increasingly greater amounts of insulin. This condition, known as insulin resistance, is a precursor to diabetes. But not only do insulin resistance and high insulin levels lead to obesity and diabetes, but the excess insulin is atherogenic. That is, it causes arterial disease and high blood pressure and can lead to a heart attack. The insulin resistance and resulting high insulin levels are now believed to be at the basis of a whole spectrum of diseases. This group of diseases has become known as Syndrome X (also more recently referred to as Metabolic Syndrome). Syndrome X includes insulin resistance, obesity (particularly abdominal obesity), high blood pressure, elevated triglycerides and small-dense LDL cholesterol, heart disease, gout, and blood clotting abnormalities.

The tests to ask for regarding Syndrome X are: Fasting Insulin Level, Fasting and 2 hr Post-Prandial Blood Glucose, and HbA1C.

For more on insulin, obesity, and heart disease, see the next chapter.

Serum Ferritin is a test that measures iron stores in the body. Excessive iron levels are potent generators of free radical activity, which will result in accelerated arterial damage and heart disease.

Toxic Metal Screen. Toxic metals very often play a role in the causation of atherosclerotic heart disease and many of the other degenerative diseases of aging. Blood levels of these metals are not adequate for evaluating the amounts in the body, as they are stored away in many organs and tissues including the bone, fat, brain, liver, thyroid, and very definitely in the heart. Some of the testing done to detect and monitor the levels of these metals (lead, mercury, cadmium, aluminum, and several others) include, hair tissue mineral analysis, and urine testing following a chelation challenge. This is done by administering a single dose, either oral, intramuscular, or intravenous, of a chelating agent and collecting a urine specimen over a measured time interval, then measuring the amounts of the toxic metals which have been excreted. See Chapter 16 on chelation therapy.

Chapter 11

Obesity and Heart Disease

We are in the midst of a major trend. People are getting fatter. Why? There is no one simple answer, but it is quite clear that we've been getting the wrong information from the food industry and the medical establishment. The low-fat message (reduce the amount of fat you eat and you will lose weight and avoid a heart attack) is not working. Actually the focus on avoiding dietary fat is finally being recognized as one of the major contributors to our epidemic of obesity. The increase in obesity in our population can be traced back to the late 1970s when the low-fat dogma began to be widely publicized. About that time, when the major organizations such as the National Institutes of Health, the American Heart Association, and the National Heart, Lung, and Blood Institute began to endorse the low-fat dogma, the food industry began to produce "low fat," "reduced fat," and "fat-free" foods. One of the big problems with that is that when fat is removed, flavor is lost. The food industry solution is to replace fat with sugar and the cheaper but even more harmful form of sugar called high fructose corn syrup.

So what's the problem? The problem is that consumption of these sugar laden fat-free foods on a day-to-day basis results in chronically elevated insulin levels and eventually insulin resistance. When the cells of the body have all the sugar they need, the excess sugar is converted to fat and the fat is stored in the fat cells. Insulin is a fat storage hormone! Excess sugar results in excess fat storage!

What else? As mentioned in the previous chapter, excess insulin is atherogenic (causes atherosclerosis, high blood pressure, and heart disease), and can eventually lead to diabetes and all of its complications. Again, this complex of maladies is called Syndrome X, and it affects a huge portion of our population.

Along with our excessive sugar consumption, we are eating more calories than ever before.

When we eat high carbohydrate, high sugar foods, our pancreas secretes insulin, which pushes sugar into our muscles and liver. For a few hours after eating a high carbohydrate meal or snack we are burning sugar for fuel and storing fat. Only after the sugar is burned up or stored as fat do insulin levels drop down. Then we start to burn fat.

High carbohydrate consumption, high insulin level, burn sugar, store fat! Low carbohydrate consumption, low insulin level, burn fat!

We want to keep our insulin levels low in order to burn fat. How do we do that? Reduce or eliminate the consumption of simple sugars like white sugar, high fructose corn syrup, honey, maple syrup, fruit juices. Eliminate white bread, and other white flour baked goods, pasta, desserts, pastries, cakes, cookies, bagels, crackers, candy, and that major health destroyer, soda pop. Increase consumption of the healthy fats as described in chapter 2. The omega 3 fats, which occur in fish, fish oil, and flax seed, will help to burn fat. Yes, you must eat fat to burn fat! You may ask, "What is left to eat if I eliminate all those foods?" Eat lots of vegetables, fruits in moderation, whole grains, eggs, lean meats (organic grass-fed if available), poultry, fish.

Soda Pop and High Fructose Corn Syrup

Because high fructose corn syrup is cheaper than sugar, it has been used as the sweetener in soda pop for the last several years. This large amount of fructose that is consumed with every serving of soda pop can only be burned for energy and saved in the liver as glycogen for later energy use in very limited amounts. The excess is converted to triglycerides which become stored as fat. The elevated triglycerides then contribute to obesity, diabetes, high blood pressure, and heart disease. Is the massive consumption of soda pop, with its large amount of high fructose corn syrup, contributing to our epidemic of obesity? I have no doubt about it. I find it distressingly common to see overweight people, young and old alike, in restaurants drinking pop with their meals. Wouldn't it make a whole lot more sense to drink water?

The artificial sweeteners are not a reasonable answer, as they also often cause very significant health problems. And according to Consumer's Research Magazine, *There is no clear-cut evidence that sugar substitutes are useful in weight reduction. On the contrary, there is some evidence that these substances may stimulate appetite.*

Aspartame (marketed as Equal and NutraSweet) is the number one source of consumer food complaints made to the FDA. Problems include seizures, headache, depression, severe confusion, loss of diabetes control, multiple sclerosis, gross weight loss or gain, accident proneness, aspartame addiction, possible causation or acceleration of Alzheimer's disease, brain tumors. Have you read about all or any of these dangers in your daily newspaper? Have you heard about them on the evening news? Why are you not hearing about this?

For more on the dangers of aspartame see www.dorway.com or www.holisticmed.com/aspartame.

Sweet Misery: A Poisoned World is a very interesting, recently made DVD which documents in a dramatic way some of the serious illnesses which are resulting from aspartame poisoning. It also investigates the political corruption which took place to allow FDA approval of this dangerous substance. This DVD is available through the website www.wnho.net. This is the website for the World Natural Health Organization.

H. J. Roberts, M.D. has been in the forefront of exposing the dangers of aspartame and the politics that keeps it on the market in spite of its appalling record of producing illness. For the whole aspartame story, I recommend his book, *Aspartame (NutraSweet): Is It Safe?*

What about **Splenda** (Sucralose)? The conclusion of an article that appears on the Sucralose Toxicity Information Center website states, *While it is unlikely that sucralose is as toxic as the poisoning that people are experiencing from Monsanto's aspartame, it is clear from the hazards seen in pre-approval research, and from its chemical structure, that years or decades of use may contribute to serious chronic immunological or neurological disorders.* See www.holisticmed.com/splenda.

Fortunately, there are a few natural very low calorie sweeteners which have no toxicity and even have health benefits. Here are two important ones.

Xylitol (also known as birch sugar) is a naturally occurring sweet compound that is found in fruits and vegetables. Studies have shown it to be valuable in the prevention of tooth decay and prevention of ear infections. It has also been proven effective in slowing stomach emptying, thus promoting a feeling of fullness with less food intake. It can be a useful sweetener for diabetics and anyone who wants a sweet taste without the negative health effects of sugar, and the artificial sweeteners.

Stevia, a natural sweetener from South America, has been used as a healthy sweetener for thousands of years. It has been proven extremely safe in numerous studies. See www.stevia.net/safety.htm.

More reasons to avoid sugar.

Our bodies were not designed to deal with the effects of the massive amounts of sugar consumed by the average American. It has been estimated that the average person consumes 140 pounds of sugar per year. And this amount continues to increase. The organs that regulate our sugar levels are stressed beyond their capacities, and every organ and cell in the body suffers as a result. The negative effects of sugar are well documented in the world's medical journals, yet the public remains pitifully uninformed.

As listed in Robert Crayhon's excellent book *Nutrition Made Simple*,

Sugar has been shown to:

- Increase the risk for breast cancer
- Double the risk for biliary tract cancer
- Deplete B vitamins and chromium
- Interfere with the absorption of calcium and magnesium
- Cause heart disease
- Increase cholesterol and insulin levels
- Raise blood pressure
- Raise triglycerides
- Weaken the immune system
- Cause a deficiency of copper

- Cause varicose veins
- Damage the kidneys
- Cause or worsen arthritis
- Cause migraine headaches
- Increase the acidity of the stomach
- Cause gallstones
- Contribute to obesity

Each of these statements is documented in the Crayhon book with references to published journal articles.

In addition to severely limiting your consumption of sugar in all its forms, you can help to keep your sugar/insulin system in balance by eating protein and fat at each meal and each snack throughout the day. By doing so, your blood sugar levels will be more stable and sugar cravings will ease off.

For very helpful information on losing weight, reversing Syndrome X, staying heart healthy, and slowing the aging process, I strongly recommend the book, *The Schwarzbein Principle* by Diana Schwarzbein, M.D.

Chapter 12

Protein

Many of us eat too little protein. Protein in optimal amounts has many benefits and is an important part of staying well. For optimal health some protein should be consumed at every meal and every snack. This will help to keep blood sugar levels balanced and energy levels up, resulting in decreased cravings for sugary high carbohydrate foods.

We get protein from lean meats, fish, seafood, eggs, tofu, and dairy products, and smaller amounts in other foods. Grains provide some protein, but are mostly starch (carbohydrate). Nuts and seeds and nut butters provide protein and are also good sources of beneficial fats.

High quality lean meats are not fattening. As a matter of fact, they are the best foods for losing excess weight. Additionally, quality meat provides several important nutrients that are either not available, or not available in significant quantity in other foods.

Some of these important nutrients are:

- Carnitine. Important for energy, particularly skeletal muscle and heart muscle energy.

- High quality protein.

- Omega 3 fatty acids (when animals graze on grasses or are fed flax seed).

- Taurine. An important amino acid that has a wide range of benefits for the heart, the eyes, and the immune system.

- Zinc. Important for immune function, brain health, and sexual function.

- Carnosine. An important anti-aging nutrient.

- Heme iron and vitamin B12. Important blood building nutrients.

- Creatine. Builds muscle mass and strength.

- CLA (conjugated linoleic acid). An anti-cancer nutrient that also helps with weight loss.

This list is adapted with modifications from the excellent book, *The Carnitine Miracle*, by Robert Crayhon, M.S., with the author's permission.

Meat has gotten a bad rap, which is undeserved. This is based on the failure to differentiate high quality meat from the meat of animals that have been raised in unnatural conditions and adulterated with toxic substances. Not all forms of meat are beneficial. High quality meat is obtained from animals that are allowed to eat the food which they are naturally inclined to eat. In the case of beef, that means that the cows have primarily grazed on grasses and have not been fed grains. The meat from those who eat grasses will be high in the beneficial omega 3 fatty acids. The meat from those fed on grains will be high in the more inflammatory omega 6 fatty acids. Ideally, the cows will not have been given hormones and antibiotics. For sources of drug-free, grass-fed beef, see the appendix.

Wild game is generally the best, most nutritious meat. Venison and wild game birds are good choices when available. Grass-fed buffalo meat is also a good choice.

The meats to avoid are the processed meats such as bologna, hot dogs, sausages, bacon, ham, cold cuts. These meat products contain nitrates, nitrites, and other preservatives, which are toxic and cancer producing. They also contain the type of cholesterol which we want to avoid, oxidized cholesterol.

- Best meat: wild game.

- Next best: organic grass fed beef, or buffalo, organic free-range chicken.

- Next: supermarket lean beef and chicken.

- Worst: processed meats.

Fish can be an excellent source of protein. The cold water fish such as salmon, mackerel, halibut and cod will also provide the important omega 3 fatty acids. A problem with much of the available fish is contamination. Mercury, PCBs and numerous other toxins that have been dumped into the lakes, rivers, and oceans accumulate in the fish and end up in our bodies when we eat the fish. Salmon, cod, mackerel, and other fish from the northern oceans are the best choices for obtaining valuable omega 3 fats and avoiding contamination. Small fish are generally less contaminated than larger fish. Particularly high in mercury contamination are tuna, swordfish, and other very large fish. See appendix for a source of uncontaminated fish high in healthful omega 3 fatty acids.

Chapter 13

Nutritional Supplements

Essential, not optional!

Perhaps your doctor or dietician has told you that supplements are not necessary, that supplements will just give you expensive urine, and that you can get all the nutrients you need from food. No study has ever been done that proves this is true. You may find it interesting that two thirds of dieticians and two thirds of cardiologists take supplements while advising their patients not to!

Most Americans go through life with many essential nutrients absent, setting themselves up for heart disease, cancer, other degenerative diseases, and either an early death or a miserable old age.

According to Robert Crayhon in his excellent book, *Nutrition Made Simple,* some of the reasons we can't get all the nutrients we need from the food that we eat are:

- Even an optimal selection of foods does not give us enough antioxidants to defend ourselves against toxic outgassing from office equipment, cigarette smoke, smog, and alcohol.

- The average person is exposed to more than five hundred chemicals in the home environment and seven hundred chemicals in drinking water that are known to deplete many nutrients.

- Soils are depleted of minerals due to chemical farming methods, acid rain, overfarming, and topsoil erosion.

- Ninety percent of us are deficient in chromium, an essential trace mineral poorly supplied by the American diet.

- Eighty percent of the carbohydrates consumed by Americans are in the form of refined flours and sugars, which are very poor sources of B6, folic acid, pantothenic acid, zinc and manganese. These nutrients are essential for health.

- The 133 pounds of sugar Americans eat each year deplete B vitamins and minerals.

- Only 9% of the population eats the recommended five servings of vitamin-rich fruits and vegetables.

- Americans eat 230 more calories per day than they did fifteen years ago. Our diet consists mostly of refined foods. Increasing our consumption of nutrient-depleted foods means we have an even higher requirement for the vitamins and minerals needed to metabolize them.

- Those who exercise regularly have a much higher need for antioxidants and minerals.

- Vitamin B2 is needed by those with hypothyroidism in amounts greater than can be found in food.

- Men and women need to be optimally nourished long before they have children.

- More than 10% of calories consumed in America come from alcoholic beverages. Alcohol depletes B vitamins, zinc, and magnesium.

- Our epidemic of degenerative diseases is caused by multiple nutrient deficiencies.

- Prescription and over-the-counter medication can deplete nutrients and create deficiencies.

- Birth control pills create vitamin B6 deficiencies and increase the need for B6 beyond what the diet can supply.

- Illness increases our need for vitamin C and zinc well beyond what food can supply.

- Millions of Americans are dieting and need supplements just to meet minimal nutrient requirements. Dieting increases free radical production, and optimal levels of antioxidants are needed to reduce damage to the liver and other organs that can occur during weight loss.

RDA versus Optimal Nutrition

The RDAs (Recommended Daily Allowances, sometimes referred to as Recommended Dietary Allowances, or more recently, Daily Reference Values) are amounts of nutrients slightly in excess of the amounts that will prevent deficiency diseases. They are far below the levels that will prevent and treat degenerative diseases like heart disease and cancer. These tiny amounts are referred to by Crayhon as "minimum wage nutrition". They are the amounts that will be adequate to prevent the deficiency diseases like scurvy, pellagra, and beri-beri. On the other hand, optimal nutrition has the potential to prevent and often reverse degenerative diseases and to promote vibrant health. You must decide if you want to make the extra effort and incur the extra expense that is required in order to enjoy vigorous health, avoid heart attacks and survive to a ripe old age. Nutritional supplements are the real treatments of choice for most of the chronic diseases that are so rampant in our modern world.

71

They are the treatments of choice because they address the real causes of our illnesses, rather than temporarily alleviating symptoms, as is done with drug therapies. For an excellent book on how to effectively treat most of our ailments with nutritional supplements, I highly recommend *Dr. Atkins' Vita-Nutrient Solution* by Robert C. Atkins, M.D.

Where to begin?

Obviously a healthful diet that includes vegetables, fruits, nuts, grass-fed meats, wild game, fish, seafood, eggs, and limited amounts of whole grains (if tolerated) is extremely important. But even a carefully planned and varied diet does not provide the optimal amounts of nutrients that will prevent heart disease and cancer and promote vigorous health and well-being.

Caveat: This chapter is not meant to be a complete coverage of the vast and important role of nutritional supplements in prevention and treatment of heart disease. For the person who is already aware of having heart disease, or who suspects heart problems, or for the person who is under treatment for heart disease or high blood pressure, it is very important to be under the care of a qualified health practitioner, preferably one who is trained in clinical nutrition in addition to having all the skills and training necessary to diagnose and treat heart disease and related problems. In the appendix are some sources to help you locate such a practitioner in your area.

Supplements for heart health

Unfortunately, many of the supplements sold in drug stores, discount stores, and even health food stores do not contain the amounts of nutrients that are stated on the labels. In fact, some are completely lacking in the stated nutrients. Additionally, serious contamination is not uncommon. More reliable sources are some of the companies who market their supplements only through health care professionals. These are referred to as professional lines of supplements. There are several such companies.

A potent multiple vitamin that contains significant amounts of all the B vitamins (enough to keep your homocysteine at a healthy low level), important minerals, and significant amounts of antioxidants will go a long way to prevent disease and help support a vigorous metabolism. This should form the foundation of your supplement program. Most of the popular multiple vitamins sold in drug stores, and advertised on TV contain amounts of nutrients that are barely adequate to prevent deficiency diseases. That is if they contain the full amounts listed on the label. Actually analysis by a panel of nutritional experts utilizing 14 different criteria and published in the excellent book, *Comparative Guide to Nutritional Supplements* by Lyle MacWilliam reveals that many popular brands contain only a small percentage of the label claim. The multiple you choose should be rich in important antioxidants, vitamin C, and vitamin E, and high in B6, folic acid and B12 to help normalize homocysteine levels. (Remember that these B vitamins are essential to keep homocysteine at healthy low levels.) It will also have significant levels of chromium, which is important in sugar and insulin metabolism, be balanced in iodine and selenium, (important for healthy thyroid function), and contain good levels of zinc for healthy immune function and protein synthesis, and boron for bone health and mental energy. If it contains alpha lipoic acid, that is a valuable bonus, as alpha lipoic acid helps to regenerate all of the other antioxidants and is itself a potent anti-oxidant. Designs for Health provides several excellent choices.

Next on the list of very important supplements is a good high potency fish oil supplement. It must be tested and found to be free of mercury and other toxic metals, PCBs and other contaminants. And it must be fresh. If it smells or tastes bad, it is rancid. Fish oil provides the very important omega 3 fatty acids, EPA (eicosapentaenoic acid) and DHA (docosahexaenoic acid). These fatty acids help the heart in many ways. They prevent blood platelets from clumping, thus avoiding abnormal clots that could cause a heart attack. Because of this effect on preventing abnormal clotting, they can be a very effective alternative to the antiquated, but still commonly used, dangerous drug, Coumadin (warfarin). These important fatty acids also lower blood pressure and help to prevent arrhythmias (irregular heart rhythm). Combined with a reduced carbohydrate intake, they will help to lower triglycerides by a very significant amount. Perhaps most importantly, the fish oils will reduce inflammation, which, as has been discussed, is believed to play a major role in heart and arterial disease. In addition to helping the heart and arteries, the fish oil supplements, by their role in reducing inflammation can be very helpful for arthritis, colitis, lung disease, auto-immune diseases, chronic fatigue syndrome, and depression. One more important point: The omega 3 fats, particularly DHA, are absolutely essential for normal development of the brain and eyes in the developing fetus, infant, and young child. The significant amounts of DHA present in breast milk provide this essential nutrient for the developing infant.

Neptune Krill Oil, an even better source of omega 3 fatty acids! The krill is a small shrimp-like crustacean that lives in abundance in the oceans, particularly in the Antarctic Ocean where the seawater is relatively pure and cold. The omega 3 fats present in krill oil occur as phospholipids, which are important natural emulsifiers. The phospholipids play many essential roles in digestion, liver function, and brain function. Because the krill oil fatty acids are integrated with the phospholipids they are efficiently and rapidly taken up by our cell membranes. Occurring naturally with these fatty acid/phospholipid complexes are some wonderful antioxidants. Because of these antioxidants, krill oil is remarkably stable and provides benefits beyond what can be expected from fish oil. The list of documented benefits from krill oil is a long one. In addition to protecting against heart attacks and strokes, its anti-inflammatory action will give relief from arthritis, nerve inflammation, asthma, and premenstrual syndrome. It supports healthy brain and liver function, helps prevent skin cancer, and increases athletic performance. Another important advantage of krill oil over fish oils: Because of its super bio-availability, it can be taken in smaller doses. Two small 500 mg soft-gels provide a full therapeutic dose.

Caveat: Krill oil should not be taken by persons allergic to shrimp. Krill oil and fish oil should not be taken prior to surgical procedures, since they have a blood thinning effect.

Magnesium is clearly the heart's most important mineral, playing a role in the function of over 300 different enzyme systems. It is estimated that 80% of Americans are deficient in magnesium. It is essential for maintaining normal heart rhythm. It plays an important role in treatment of high blood pressure, can decrease frequency of angina pectoris (chest pain) episodes, and it helps to prevent abnormal blood clots. These are just a few of the many roles that magnesium plays in maintaining healthy heart and blood vessel function. One difficulty with supplementation of magnesium is that it is irritating to the intestinal tract and often is poorly absorbed. For that reason, complementary alternative physicians often administer it intravenously. One of the best absorbed and least irritating <u>oral</u> forms of magnesium is called Magnesium Glycinate Chelate. It is manufactured by Albion Labs, the world leader in manufacture of chelated minerals, and sold through health care practitioners.

Beyond the basics

There are many other important nutrients to enhance heart function and prevent heart attacks. Here are some of the important ones utilized by nutritionally aware health practitioners.

CoEnzyme Q 10 (CoQ10) is one of the most important nutrients for healthy heart function. It is a necessary substance for the heart to maintain its continuous energy output. And we don't get much in our food. Organ meats are the main source in our food supply, and most people don't consume many of these. Much research has been done on the role of CoQ10 in prevention and treatment of various heart ailments. It is very well documented to improve the function of the heart in the increasingly common condition known as congestive heart failure. This is the condition where the heart muscle contractions have become too weak to adequately pump the blood through the arteries. Fluid builds up in the lungs and throughout the body, resulting in severe breathing difficulties and generalized weakness. While standard medical practitioners use drugs to treat this condition, the drugs have limited usefulness if the all-important CoQ10 and other needed nutritional factors are not supplied. In addition to being very important for treatment of congestive heart failure, CoQ10 can play an important role in the treatment of angina pectoris (chest pain), arrhythmias, mitral valve prolapse, and high blood pressure. Other non-cardiac benefits of CoQ10 are enhanced immune function, and improved gum health. Recent research has also demonstrated benefit of high dose CoQ10 for Parkinson's Disease.

For people taking statin drugs, it is especially important to take CoQ10. In chapter 6 we discussed the well established dangerous suppression of the liver's production of CoQ10 by the statin drugs, which is believed to be playing a role in the current epidemic of congestive heart failure. For those who are inclined to be part of the statin drug experiment, a moderate daily dose of CoQ10 will allow you to avoid this severe statin side effect. It will not, however, save you from the many other potentially dangerous side effects of the statin drugs.

CoQ10 is a lipid soluble (fat soluble) substance which is somewhat difficult to absorb and utilize. CoQ10 powder, or capsules containing powder, should be taken with a fatty food, such as olive oil, butter, flax oil or peanut butter to enhance absorption. An even better way to enhance absorption of the powdered form of CoQ10 is to place the powder into a hot cup of liquid such as tea or coffee with cream or butter added. The combination of heat and fat produce ideal conditions for enhancing absorption. Emulsified forms of CoQ10 in a softgel are available and are better absorbed. CoQ10 that is emulsified in rice bran oil and stabilized with beeswax is an excellent choice.

Carnitine is an important nutrient for healthy heart function. Our bodies can make carnitine, but not in the quantities that will help to maintain optimal health. Its main function is to increase energy by enhancing the burning of fat. Since the heart uses fat as its main fuel, carnitine is essential for efficient heart function. It also plays an important role in weight loss. Studies have shown that carnitine can significantly reduce complications following a heart attack. Since it is converting fat into energy, the person taking carnitine will generally feel more energetic. It greatly enhances exercise performance. These are just a few of the benefits of this amazing nutrient. For the whole story, I suggest the excellent Robert Crayhon book, *The Carnitine Miracle*. A recently published study from Australia demonstrated that carnitine outperformed testosterone in dealing with male aging issues, including depression and sexual dysfunction. The preferred form of carnitine is carnitine tartrate. It can be taken as a pleasant tasting powder dissolved in water, or in capsule form.

Taurine is a multi-faceted nutrient that can play multiple roles in the <u>treatment</u> of heart disease, in addition to its valuable role in heart disease <u>prevention</u>. One of its important functions is to help keep magnesium and potassium inside of our cells while keeping sodium on the outside. In this way it acts as a diuretic, but without any of the side effects of the chemical diuretics. For arrhythmias (disturbances of heart rhythm), many nutritionally aware physicians consider the combination of taurine and magnesium as the treatment of choice. While helping to maintain normal rhythm, it also strengthens the heart's contractions and helps to normalize blood pressure. Taurine is often very helpful in controlling seizure disorders. It is known also to be helpful for warding off asthma attacks, and is reported to be an important nutrient for prevention and treatment of macular degeneration, the serious retinal disease that is the main cause of blindness in elderly people.

Hawthorn is an herb which functions in a way similar to digitalis in the control of heart rhythm and heart failure, but without any of the side-effects commonly seen with the drug. It also reduces elevated blood pressure, enhances blood flow through the coronary arteries, and relieves inflammation. It is widely used by nutritionally aware physicians for any and all heart related problems.

Vitamin E has been used by ever increasing numbers of people since the 1950s for its value as an antioxidant and for its benefits in cardiovascular disease, cancer prevention, lung protection, relief of menopausal symptoms, vision protection, and immune enhancement. In recent years its value in reducing the incidence of heart attacks has been documented by several large-scale studies. The vitamin E complex consists of tocopherols and tocotrienols. Within the vitamin E complex, there are four tocopherol fractions and four tocotrienol fractions. Until recently, it has been believed that the fraction called d-alpha tocopherol is the most important active principle. However, recent research reveals that gamma tocopherol is the more effective antioxidant free radical scavenger. The gamma fraction has also been found to have anti-inflammatory activity, which we know is important for the prevention and control of arterial disease. **Important message:** The vitamin E that you take should be vitamin E complex, high in gamma tocopherol. The synthetic vitamin E which is commonly sold in drug stores, grocery stores, discount stores and in some health food stores is worthless. Check the label! You can recognize the synthetic version by the words, **dl**-alpha tocopherol or **dl**-alpha tocopheryl acetate or succinate. Don't waste your money on these synthetics.

Beyond Vitamin E, a safe alternative to statin drugs.

The tocotrienols, which formerly were considered relatively unimportant components of the vitamin E complex have recently been recognized as extremely valuable nutrients for treatment of cardiovascular disease, and, in fact, are considered by some researchers to be 40 to 60 times more powerful than the other vitamin E components at protecting our cells from oxidative damage. **Annatto Tocotrienols**, a product developed by nutritional researcher Barrie Tan, Ph.D., and marketed by Designs for Health is a small softgel that contains only the gamma and delta tocotrienols. These fractions, when isolated from the other components of the vitamin E complex take on a powerful therapeutic role that addresses many of the factors involved in the development of atherosclerotic heart disease. Recent research demonstrates that these tocotrienol fractions inhibit the liver's synthesis of cholesterol, but, unlike the statin drugs, they do not inhibit its production of CoQ10. This results in lowered serum cholesterol, lowered LDL, slightly elevated HDL, and lowered triglycerides. Most importantly, these tocotrienol fractions inhibit inflammation, prevent platelet clumping (to prevent abnormal clots), prevent vasoconstriction (blood vessel narrowing), and prevent the stickiness that promotes arterial plaque build-up (adhesion molecule activity). Actually, the therapeutic profile of **Annatto Tocotrienols** is similar to that of the statin drugs, but without any of the dangerous side effects. The amount of cholesterol lowering from this supplement is not nearly as dramatic as that seen with the statin drugs. But we have learned that the benefit to be gained from the statins, if any, is due to its other properties, not due to its lowering of cholesterol.

Anti-inflammatory herbs and enzymes. To help prevent and reverse the chronic inflammation that is a component of arterial disease, and which is signaled by an elevation of the C-reactive protein blood test, a natural approach utilizing combinations of herbs, bioflavonoids, and proteolytic enzymes which target the metabolic pathways of the inflammatory response can be an effective therapy in conjunction with the important dietary and lifestyle changes previously discussed. Some of these substances which can be used to favorably and powerfully modify the inflammatory response include boswellia, turmeric, ginger, quercetin, rutin, rosemary, resveratrol, in addition to certain proteolytic enzymes. These products can be used safely and without side effects to inhibit all kinds of inflammatory conditions. This is in contrast to the commonly used anti-inflammatory drugs, all of which carry the risk of serious side effects.

These are a few of the important nutrients that are available in supplement form that can be utilized as part of a holistic program to prevent, treat, and often reverse heart and artery disease. As stated previously, when disease is present, it is very important to be under the care of a qualified health care practitioner.

Vitamin C, Lysine, and Proline. The Linus Pauling-Matthias Rath Heart Therapy. This therapy has so much potential for prevention, treatment and reversal of heart disease that I have devoted a separate chapter to it. See Chapter 17.

Supplement Source. Over the years I have utilized the supplements of several excellent companies that sell their nutrients only through health care professionals. I have seen analyses of many of the over-the-counter supplements that are sold in drug stores, discount stores, and health food stores. A few check out very well. Many others, including some that are sold through health care practitioners are a disgrace, in terms of contamination and lack of stated potency. On the other hand, I know that the quality control, potency, and purity provided by the Designs for Health company is as good as it gets. The folks at Designs for Health are extremely ethical, and are right on top of the latest nutritional science. They continue to come out with new cutting-edge nutritional products when there is good science to support such products. See the appendix of this book for information on how your nutritionally oriented health care practitioner can purchase the Designs for Health supplements for your health enhancement program.

Chapter 14

Complementary Alternative Medicine-Integrative Medicine

At this time in the history of modern medicine, we are in the midst of a massive paradigm shift. The public and, finally, a very significant minority of physicians have become aware that the focus of the medical profession throughout most of the 20th century and into the 21st on pharmaceutical treatment of disease, to the forced exclusion of natural methods of healing, is not productive of good health for the individual or the nation. The idea of making war on various diseases by the introduction and seductive marketing of a continuous profusion of ever more toxic and increasingly expensive drugs is producing a population of drug-dependent sick people, and is, in fact, bankrupting our economy.

Fortunately there are now many physicians who are stepping away from the constraints of conventional mainstream medicine, whose focus is on helping their patients achieve optimal wellness, as opposed to simply prescribing a series of toxic drugs. The field of medical practice which includes these practitioners has become known as integrative medicine, complementary alternative medicine, holistic medicine, or simply, alternative medicine. Nutritional intervention is only one of the many modalities utilized by these practitioners to help the patient heal himself. But nutrition is universally recognized as one of the basic pillars of healing. Also integral to the concept of alternative medicine is that healing, to be effective, implies that the patient must become actively involved in the healing process. He (or she) must take responsibility for changing the life-style and dietary mistakes that have caused him(or her) to veer from the path of wellness to the path of disease. The patient must be the healer. The physician, hopefully, will guide him (or her) along the path.

From simple prevention to treatment of life-threatening illness, nutritional therapies play a most important role. In the last quarter century there has been an explosion of research published in medical and research journals throughout the world, documenting what many forward thinking practitioners have known through clinical experience and just plain common sense. For treatment of disease, nutritional and other natural therapies work as well as, or usually better than drugs, and without any dangerous side effects. And, of course, for prevention of disease, drugs, by their very nature, are of no value whatsoever.

Stress

One of the important aspects of an integrated approach to health care is to help the patient learn to control excessive stress. Stress causes the release of adrenalin and cortisol from the adrenal glands, (the fight or flight response). This is a normal response and is essential for our survival. These hormones mobilize sugar into the blood stream, triggering a rise in insulin to take sugar into our cells and to our brain where we need it for quick action. Stress also triggers the hormones called eicosanoids, which are involved with clotting of blood. However, excess stress can produce excess clotting, which can contribute to heart attacks. When stress is prolonged, as it often is in this highly competitive world that we live in, it can lead to chronic high insulin levels and insulin resistance, which will promote arterial plaque and heart attacks. Excess stress is a major contributor to heart attacks, and effectively reducing stress is an important part of the get well and avoid heart attack equation.

Exercise

Exercise on a daily basis will play multiple roles in improving heart function and preventing heart attacks. Exercise must be appropriate to the person's physical condition. Even as little exercise as walking 10 minutes a day has been documented to help reduce stress, strengthen heart activity, reduce blood pressure, and help digestive functions. On the other hand, extreme exercise without adequate anti-oxidant protection produces excess free radical activity, which can lead to more plaque formation, platelet stickiness, and higher risk for heart attack. Very strenuous exercise creates a need for higher levels of antioxidants. A person with existing heart disease should only do strenuous exercise under the guidance of a physician, and perhaps with a fitness trainer.

Drugs versus Nutrients (Blockers versus Enablers)

As expressed by the late Robert Atkins, M.D. in his excellent book, *Dr. Atkins' Vita-Nutrient Solution*, drugs and nutrients can sometimes accomplish many of the same things. However, drugs accomplish their effects by blocking some process in the body, usually an enzyme, whereas, nutrients enable the body to do what it needs to do by enhancing a natural physiologic process.

Nutrients usually accomplish their benefits slowly over a long period of time. Drugs work much more rapidly, and thus can be very important in acute situations. The complementary alternative physician utilizes the best of what is available for his patient's particular situation. Sometimes that will include drugs in addition to natural healing therapies. Obviously the treatment of choice should be the one which achieves the desired therapeutic effect with the least damage. When there is a choice, nutrition should always be preferred to drug therapies. Often in dealing with a patient who has been under treatment by conventional physicians, one who decides to change from the path of disease treatment toward the path of seeking wellness and optimal health, the main challenge, for the alternative physician, will be to carefully wean the patient off the multitude of unnecessary toxic medications that have been prescribed for symptoms, but which are now producing a whole new set of problems because of the inherent toxicity of all drugs.

Prevention versus Treatment

Most of the preventive nutritional strategies described in this book can be undertaken without professional help. However, if significant disease is diagnosed or suspected, or if symptoms such as chest pain, shortness of breath, or leg pain on walking are present, or if any other troubling symptoms are persistent, it is imperative that a competent health practitioner be involved in your care. See the appendix of this book for organizations that will help you find a qualified practitioner in your area.

Chapter 15

The Low Thyroid-Heart Disease Connection

The late Broda Barnes, M.D., a pioneer in the prevention of heart disease, dedicated more than 50 years of his life to researching, discovering, and treating thyroid disease. Through much research and the treating of many thousands of patients, he gained valuable insight into the connections between thyroid disease and many other disease conditions, including atherosclerotic heart disease. Through his books and teachings, he was able to share his discoveries with numerous physicians to the benefit of many of their patients throughout the world.

One of his many significant discoveries was that the reliance of most physicians on thyroid function blood tests for the diagnosis of hypothyroidism (under-activity of the thyroid gland), left many patients with the condition undiagnosed. Because of the medical profession's steadfast dependency on blood tests, many of their patients continued to suffer the debilitating symptoms of hypothyroidism and its related conditions for the rest of their lives. Sad to say, this situation persists to this day.

He observed also, that patients who took natural dessicated thyroid (from an animal source) as thyroid replacement therapy got significantly better relief of their symptoms than those who took the synthetic thyroid pills. Most physicians who are open-minded enough to consider using the natural thyroid replacement (dessicated thyroid) agree that they see significantly better results than can be obtained by the synthetic thyroid.

Some of the many symptoms of hypothyroidism are fatigue, lethargy, constipation, dry skin, dry coarse hair, facial and generalized puffiness, slow heart rate, menstrual disorders, low sex drive, sluggish mental functioning, forgetfulness, depression, cold hands and feet, thinning of eyebrows, elevated cholesterol, sometimes high blood pressure, cold intolerance, and low body temperature.

Dr. Barnes developed the basal body temperature test to help him verify the diagnosis when the clinical signs and symptoms suggested hypothyroidism. This simply involves checking and recording your body temperature in the morning on awakening for several days. A low body temperature suggests hypothyroidism.

I found, in my practice, that discovering and treating this condition by the Barnes method was one of the simplest and yet most rewarding experiences of my career. Through the taking of this tiny one-a-day tablet, many patients made major life-changing improvements in their health. I was pleased to occasionally receive referrals from Dr. Barnes when patients in my area were in need of someone who understood the Broda Barnes concepts of thyroid disease.

But the important point for the reader of this book who wants to prevent heart attacks is that Dr. Barnes elucidated a connection between hypothyroidism and coronary artery disease (heart disease). He discovered and wrote about this many years ago, and it is only now beginning to be recognized by the medical profession. He observed over a period of many years with thousands of patients, that his patients who were receiving adequate thyroid replacement therapy did not have heart attacks.

Here's why. Excess free radicals cause areas of inflammation and microscopic tissue death. When the body attempts to repair these injuries it forms scar tissue utilizing cholesterol (remember that it is a repair substance). Cholesterol and calcium are deposited in the scar tissue to form atherosclerotic plaque. Antioxidants, including those that are produced within the body are attempting to stop this free radical activity. When thyroid hormone levels are inadequate, the endogenous (produced by the body) anti-oxidant activity is slowed down. This allows the atherosclerotic process to proceed more rapidly. Also, when thyroid activity is low, the immune functions are sluggish, resulting in impaired ability to fight off infections. Infections create inflammation, which accelerates the atherosclerotic process.

So, discovering and treating under-activity of thyroid function can be a very important part of preventing heart and arterial disease. Remember that in many cases of hypothyroidism the blood tests cannot be relied upon. Hypothyroidism is a very common condition. Dr. Barnes estimated that it occurs in 40% of the population. Most of these cases are never diagnosed. If you suspect that you have hypothyroidism because you suffer from some of the above described symptoms, you may have to search for a physician who is not locked into the notion that the condition can only be diagnosed by blood tests.

For more information on this important subject, read *Hypothyroidism, The Unsuspected Illness* and *Solved, the Riddle of Heart Disease*, both by Broda Barnes, M.D. The Broda Barnes Research Foundation website can be found at www.brodabarnes.org. The foundation makes these books available and can supply a list of practitioners who utilize the Broda Barnes concepts in their practices.

Chapter 16

Chelation Therapy

It would not be appropriate for me to write a book on non-toxic safe prevention and treatment of heart disease without discussing this most valuable, yet largely unrecognized, treatment.

As an essential part of my practice for more than 15 years, I have seen intravenous chelation therapy work near miracles on far advanced cases of heart and blood vessel disease, including saving the limbs of patients who were scheduled for amputation due to gangrene caused by major circulation impairment and diabetes. Saving patients from the need for heart bypass surgery is a common occurrence among the innovative and courageous physicians who utilize this safe and effective, but "politically incorrect," treatment. The treatment involves intravenous administration of a synthetic amino acid called ethylene diamine tetra-acetic acid (EDTA) in a solution which also contains important nutrients. The intravenous solution is repeated approximately 2 or 3 times per week until a series of 20, 30, 40 or more IVs have been given. The EDTA in this solution binds with and removes from the body, toxic metals and calcium that has been deposited in the atherosclerotic plaques of arteries. The result is vastly improved metabolism of all the enzyme systems in the body, (which were being poisoned by toxic metal burden), and improved circulation through all the arteries. Blood flow improves through the coronary arteries in the heart, resulting in improved heart function, and through the carotid arteries to the brain. This improved circulation and improved metabolic function, in a very real sense, effects a true reversal of the aging process. Chest pains due to impaired coronary artery circulation disappear, memory and thinking processes improve, walking becomes easier, sexual function improves.

Chelation therapy was first utilized in the 1950s, and has been given to many hundreds of thousands of patients with a remarkable record of effectiveness and safety. Numerous studies, both published and unpublished establish the effectiveness of chelation therapy at approximately 85%. Most of the small percentage of patients who fail to improve are those who fail to give up their toxic lifestyles, particularly the smoking of cigarettes. Chelating physicians expect their patients to adopt all the important dietary and lifestyle habits that constitute a holistic approach.

To learn more about this valuable therapy, I highly recommend the book written by Terry Chappell, M.D. called *Questions From the Heart: Answers to 100 Questions About Chelation Therapy, a Safe Alternative to Bypass Surgery*. There are several other good books on the subject, and some are listed in the appendix to this book. To find a physician in your area who is qualified to administer chelation therapy, call the American College of Advancement in Medicine (ACAM) at 800-532-3688 or check the websites of ACAM, www.ACAM.com, or the International College of Integrative Medicine (www.ICIMED.com).

Chapter 17

Linus Pauling-Matthias Rath Heart Therapy

One of the true geniuses of science of the 20th century, Linus Pauling, Ph.D. (1901-1995) was the only person to be awarded two unshared Nobel prizes. The first was for his research into the nature of the chemical bond, and the second for his efforts toward achieving world peace. His hundreds of groundbreaking discoveries and his efforts to end war have had a profound influence on all humankind. However, when he became interested in vitamin C (ascorbic acid) and the common cold, the medical establishment labeled him a quack. When he claimed, based on clinical studies, that vitamin C had value in prevention and treatment of cancer, he really incurred the wrath of the medical and scientific community and became a medical pariah.

In the last 2 decades of his life, working with his associate, Dr. Matthias Rath, he focused his attention on prevention and treatment of heart disease. It now appears that his approach, in which he considered heart disease to be a form of chronic scurvy (vitamin C deficiency), may provide a simple solution to the scourge that has baffled scientists and medical researchers for the past one hundred years.

Scurvy was initially observed during the 15th and 16th centuries. On long sea voyages the British sailors developed listlessness, bleeding gums, bruising, weight loss, painful muscles, swollen painful joints, and loss of teeth. After many years of suffering and many deaths, it was discovered that the disease could be cured by consuming limes. Eventually limes were routinely administered to the British sailors to prevent the condition. Hence, they became known as "Limeys." It took many more years for science to realize that vitamin C was necessary for the formation of collagen, the fibrous protein material that makes up the bulk of the connective tissue of the body, including the skin, bones, ligaments, cartilage, and importantly, the arteries, and that scurvy was the result of its absence. Full-blown scurvy is seen far less often in modern times, although it does occur when fresh vegetables and fruit are absent from the diet, as they often are these days, particularly among the elderly.

What Pauling realized, through keen observation and careful research, is that a less intense chronic form of vitamin C deficiency is the underlying cause of atherosclerotic heart disease, and many of the other chronic degenerative diseases that plague our aging population.

The observation that animals, other than humans, guinea pigs, and certain primates, do not suffer from atherosclerotic heart disease, was one of the considerations that led to the suspicion that heart disease is related to a lack of adequate amounts of vitamin C in the blood stream. All other animals, those who do not develop heart disease, make vitamin C in their bodies. Cats, dogs, pigs, and most other animals are able to wallow in filth and be exposed to all kinds of infectious organisms, and still remain in relatively good health. This is because they make their own vitamin C in rather massive amounts. Somewhere along the way, through millions of years of evolution, we humans lost the ability to do that. We cannot make even one molecule of this extremely important vitamin.

Dr. G. C. Willis, a Canadian physician, observed during the 1950s that atherosclerotic plaques form over vitamin C deficient arterial tissues in both guinea pigs and humans. He also found that these plaques build up in areas where the arteries are most bent and squeezed. Additional studies by others during the same time period revealed that tissues of patients who suffer from heart disease are significantly depleted of vitamin C. Willis determined that the body was laying down plaque to strengthen these areas of the arteries that were weakened by lack of vitamin C and mechanical stress.

During the 1980s several important discoveries took place, which made possible the eventual development of the Pauling-Rath Therapy for Heart Disease, otherwise known as Lp(a) Binding Inhibitor Therapy. Pauling and his associate Matthias Rath, M.D. utilized the knowledge that the Lipoprotein(a) molecule (discovered around 1964) was involved in the laying down of plaque. Another important piece of the puzzle fell into place about that time when it was discovered that the Lp(a) molecule has "lysine binding sites."

The theory goes like this: Because vitamin C is absolutely vital for the health and strength of the arteries, the human being, lacking high levels of vitamin C in the blood stream, begins to develop lesions (small cracks) in the lining of the arteries at stress points. Within these cracks are lysine strands. The liver, sensing a lack of adequate vitamin C, generates increasing levels of Lp(a), a sticky artery repair substance. Having lysine binding sites as part of their structure, the Lp(a) molecules seek out lysine. Finding lysine strands in the bruised or cracked arterial wall, they attach to the wall at the site of the bruise. This is the body's repair mechanism. Dr. Rath has described it as similar to a plaster cast reinforcing the weak arterial wall. In the continued absence of adequate levels of vitamin C, the process goes beyond repair and begins to build up excessive amounts of plaque, which eventually obstruct the flow of blood and lead to all the problems we know as atherosclerotic heart disease. It could be said that Lp(a) based plaques were an evolutionary counter-measure for the chronic low levels of vitamin C in human beings. As expressed by Rath and

Pauling, Lp(a) operates in the blood as a surrogate for vitamin C. Lysine is an essential amino acid and a required building block of proteins.

The solution

The elegant and yet rather simple solution devised by Drs. Pauling and Rath is to take amounts of vitamin C on a daily basis that will approach the levels that are equivalent to what most lower animals make. This allows the body to form collagen, which is necessary for arterial strength, flexibility, and healing. Also fairly large amounts of lysine taken daily will bind with the Lp(a) binding sites, effectively neutralizing the Lp(a). This Lp(a), now rendered harmless, will cease building up on the arterial wall.

To quote Dr. Pauling: *Knowing that lysyl (lysine) residues (in the arterial wall) are what cause Lp(a) to get stuck to the wall of the artery and form atherosclerotic plaques, any physical chemist would say at once that the thing to do is prevent that by putting the amino acid lysine in the blood to a greater extent than it is normally. Lysine is essential for life. You have to get about one gram a day to keep in protein balance, but you can take lysine, pure lysine, a perfectly nontoxic substance in food, as pills, which puts extra lysine molecules in the blood. They enter into competition with the lysyl residues on the wall of arteries and, accordingly, act to prevent Lp(a) from being deposited, or even will work to pull it loose and destroy atherosclerotic plaques.* Linus Pauling, Journal of Optimum Nutrition, August 1994.

As the levels of vitamin C and lysine are maintained over a period of time, the vitamin C increases collagen production and improves the strength and health of the arteries, and the lysine prevents plaque build-up, and eventually dissolves existing plaque.

The dose of vitamin C required to prevent chronic scurvy and the heart disease that is a part of it is between 3000 and 10,000 mg. per day. The dose of lysine recommended by Pauling is between 2000 and 6000 mg. per day. He referred to the two substances as Lp(a) binding inhibitors.

Pauling himself took 18,000 mg. of vitamin C per day, reasoning that some of the ingested amount would not be absorbed, and that it is far better to take too much than not enough. Both vitamin C and lysine are extremely safe. The only possible side effect of vitamin C is loose bowels if the bowel tolerance dose is exceeded. It is best to start with a small amount, and gradually increase to the therapeutic dose.

More recently, proline, another amino acid has been found to be an effective Lp(a) binding inhibitor, perhaps more effective than lysine. Since the Lp(a) molecule has both lysine binding sites and proline binding sites, 250 mg. to 2000 mg. of proline are now recommended to be added to the protocol. Proline is a non-essential amino acid that also plays an important role in protein synthesis.

Ascorbate, the Science of Vitamin C by Steve Hickey, Ph.D. and Hilary Roberts, Ph.D. is a new book (published 2004) that provides the most complete and up-to-date evaluation of all the research on vitamin C. I highly recommend this book to anyone with a serious interest in this most amazing and important nutrient. In a completely unbiased manner and in a highly readable style, they summarize and analyze all the research, both positive and negative, on the role of vitamin C in heart disease, cancer, infections, and in the maintenance of good health. In regard to heart disease they also discuss the role of tocotrienols and other antioxidants. Regarding the Pauling-Rath therapy and the evidence to support it, they find some fault with the Pauling-Rath concept of LP(a) in plaque formation, but basically agree that there is much scientific support for the concept that heart disease is a form of chronic scurvy. The problem is that the early research, done at the test-tube level and the experimental animal level has never been followed through in the form of properly structured clinical studies on human beings. The clinical studies that have been done have all been carried out with doses far too low to produce the expected clinical results. The animal studies, however, have been replicated and validated. In animals, heart disease can be caused by lack of vitamin C and reversed by supplying it. The relationship between antioxidants and plaque in animals is established.

The medical establishment, in its zeal to continue promoting the cholesterol/heart disease connection has failed in its obligation to follow up this extremely promising therapy. The basic experiments that could have validated this simple and inexpensive treatment for heart disease have just not been done. How many hundreds of thousands of lives might have been saved over these past 50 years?

The hero of this part of the story is Dr. Matthias Rath, who in the face of total resistance on the part of the medical establishment has conducted an amazing crusade to get the truth out regarding these simple solutions to the world's leading killer diseases. He has written several books, lectured throughout the world to both professional and lay audiences, and is using the profits from his book sales to continue research on these therapies.

I want to give thanks and credit to researcher, Owen Fonorow, Ph.D. for providing much of the information in this chapter.

For more information on the Pauling-Rath Therapy for Heart Disease I recommend the following websites:

- www.thecureforheartdisease.com
- www.vitamincfoundation.org

Dr. Matthias Rath's web site is:

- www.dr-rath-research.org

Chapter 18

Summary

You've been told that:

- Cholesterol is your enemy.

- It will clog your arteries and cause a heart attack.

- It is a major cause of heart disease.

- Taking drugs to suppress the level of cholesterol in your blood is a logical, reasonable, and safe way to avoid a heart attack.

However, by reading this book, you have learned that:

- Cholesterol is an extremely important molecule for a healthy fully functional body.

- The cholesterol that you eat has little or no effect on the cholesterol level in your blood.

- When you eat less cholesterol your body will make more to compensate.

- Elevated cholesterol levels are only one risk factor among many that are <u>sometimes</u> associated with heart attacks, and that at least half of all heart attacks occur in people who have "normal" or low cholesterol levels.

- The things that cause heart disease (such as smoking, sedentary life style, obesity, excessive sugar and other refined carbohydrate consumption, trans fats, lack of essential nutrients) also cause elevated cholesterol levels. But the diet/cholesterol/heart disease zealots have confused <u>association</u> with <u>causation</u>.

- The lipid hypothesis, on which modern medicine relies in its efforts to reduce heart attacks is based on faulty research, by biased researchers who most often have gained financially by producing study results that have helped to promote pharmaceutical sales.

- Studies which have showed slight improvement in heart attack statistics by lowering cholesterol with drugs have also shown increased deaths from cancer, strokes, suicides, and accidents.

- The heavily promoted statin drugs used to reduce cholesterol levels are producing an epidemic of congestive heart failure in addition to a host of other side effects, ranging from minor symptoms, to serious memory failure, to severe muscle pain, liver disease, kidney disease and death.

On the other hand, you've also learned that:

- There are safe and effective alternative ways to reduce your risk of having a heart attack. You've learned how to choose healthy fats and avoid toxic "bad" fats.

- Cholesterol and other elevated lipid levels will normalize naturally when the dietary and lifestyle causative factors are eliminated and the important missing nutrients are supplied.

- There are many experienced, well-trained physicians and other practitioners who can help you to enjoy better health, prevent heart attacks, and if needed provide scientifically proven non-drug treatments for heart and blood vessel disease.

My hope is that I have been able to open your eyes to the huge health potential which awaits the open-minded reader in the vast universe of natural health care and integrative complementary alternative medicine.

Health is not to be found within the multi-billion dollar disease care industry. This industry, with its multi-national pharmaceutical giants, hospital conglomerates, and HMO type disease care plans, its legions of physicians robotically prescribing the latest toxic, over-priced, over-hyped drugs, relies on a constant supply of sick patients for its very existence. Simple inexpensive solutions to staying healthy are not welcome. The disease care industry is on a fast track toward bankrupting the nation.

If you are to avoid heart disease and lead a long healthy life, you must take the initiative. When you are living a healthy life style, avoiding toxins, eating a healthy diet, and supplying your body with the important nutrients described in this book, you can

Stop Worrying About Cholesterol!

Avoid a Heart Attack and Live a Long Healthy Life!

Epilogue

New 2004 Guidelines for Selling More Statin Drugs! Skullduggery at the National Institutes of Health?

In July 2004 the National Cholesterol Education Program, which is a division of the National Institutes of Health issued new blood cholesterol guidelines. These guidelines are endorsed by the American Heart Association and the American College of Cardiology and, thus, will become part of the practices of most of the physicians throughout the United States.

The previous target of 100 mg/dl of LDL "bad cholesterol" was not low enough. Now, based on new research findings, doctors are being encouraged to reduce their high-risk patients' LDL to 70.

The **2001** guidelines were referred to by Uffe Ravnskov, M.D. as *New Guidelines, for Converting Healthy People into Patients.* In his thoughtful essay by that title he exposed the irrationality, bias, and conflict of interest in the promulgation of these guidelines which made many millions more people candidates for statin drugs.

Prior to the 2001 guidelines, approximately 13 million Americans were taking statin drugs. Responding to the 2001 NIH guidelines, doctors increased their prescribing of these dangerous drugs to the extent that some 36 million are now taking them, resulting in current sales of about $20 billion per year.

With the new **2004** guidelines, Dr. James Cleeman, coordinator of the National Cholesterol Education Program, estimates that an additional 7 million people will be taking statin drugs.

We can be certain that the increased doses of these potent drugs that will be required to achieve the newly recommended lower levels of blood cholesterol will result in significant increases in the number and severity of adverse effects. Lots more muscle pain, liver disease, rhabdomyolysis (severe muscle deterioration, which sometimes results in kidney failure and death). Yes, more depression and anxiety, memory impairment, mental confusion, more transient global amnesia. More infections, particularly in the elderly, where higher cholesterol levels are protective against infection. More heart failure, and probably, in years to come, more cancer. And, of course, lots more visits to doctors offices, hospitals, and pharmacies. Huge increases in medical costs, and of course, many more billions of dollars for the pharmaceutical companies.

As if these new guidelines were not broad enough, Dr. Cleeman stated that these guideline updates may not be the final word on LDL goals. Three ongoing trials could lead to even broader recommendations.

Could there be something behind the releasing of these new guidelines other than a desire to reduce the incidence of heart disease?

Should we follow the money?

Shortly after the release of the new 2004 guidelines, Newsday, a Long Island, NY newspaper reported that some of the expert panelists who decided these guidelines had ties to the pharmaceutical industry. Surprise? There was a call to the National Cholesterol Education Panel for disclosure. This is what was revealed.

Out of nine panelists:

- Seven have financial connections to Pfizer, manufacturer of the cholesterol lowering drug, Lipitor, the largest selling drug in the world.

- Five have served as consultants to Pfizer.

- Seven have financial connections to Merck, manufacturer of Zocor, another huge-selling cholesterol lowering drug.

- Only one panelist has no financial connections to any drug company.

- Eight of the panelists have received research grants or honoraria (payment) for speaking engagements at meetings designed to promote cholesterol lowering drugs.

Does this look like conflict of interest? Can we expect unbiased opinions in the face of such massive conflict of interest?

What do you think?

On September 23, 2004 a petition was submitted by The Center for Science in the Public Interest to the National Institutes of Health seeking an independent review panel to re-evaluate the new National Cholesterol Education Program guidelines. It challenged the conclusions which led to the new guidelines on both a scientific and a conflict-of-interest basis. It was signed by 35 prestigious scientists, most of whom are affiliated with major universities.

Noting that *The vast majority of heart disease can be prevented by adapting healthy habits,* the final paragraph of the petition states: *The American people are poorly served when government-sanctioned clinical recommendations, uncritically amplified by the media, misdirect attention and resources to expensive medical therapies that may not be scientifically justified. Only an independent review, totally free from conflicts of interest, can restore public confidence by determining if that has happened in this case. We therefore request that you move expeditiously to appoint such a panel and provide it with the resources needed to conduct the review.*

Appendix

Books

Ravnskov, Uffe, M.D. *The Cholesterol Myths: Exposing the Fallacy that Saturated Fat and Cholesterol cause Heart Disease.*

McCully, Kilmer S., M.D. *The Heart Revolution: The Extraordinary Discovery That Finally Laid the Cholesterol Myth to Rest.*

Graveline, Duane, M.D. *Lipitor, Thief of Memory: Statin Drugs and the Misguided War on Cholesterol.*

Crayhon, Robert, M.S. *Nutrition Made Simple, A Comprehensive Guide to the Latest Findings in Optimal Nutrition.*

Crayhon, Robert, M.S. *The Carnitine Miracle: The Supernutrient Program That Promotes High Energy, Fat Burning, Heart Health, Brain Wellness and Longevity.*

Erasmus, Udo, Ph.D. *Fats and Oils: The Complete Guide to Fats and Oils in Health and Nutrition.*

Schwarzbein, Diana, M.D. *The Schwarzbein Principle: The Truth About Losing Weight, Being Healthy, and Feeling Younger.*

Schwarzbein, Diana, M.D., Deville, Nancy, and Jacob Jaffe, Evelyn *The Schwarzbein Principle Cookbook.*

Atkins, Robert, M.D. *Dr. Atkins' Vita-Nutrient Solution: Nature's Answer to Drugs.*

Fallon, Sally, Enig, Mary, Ph.D. and Connolly, Pat *Nourishing Traditions.*

Chappell, Terry, M.D. *Questions from the Heart: Answers to 100 Questions about Chelation Therapy, a Safe Alternative to Bypass Surgery.*

Walker, Morton, D.P.M. *The Chelation Way: The Complete Book of Chelation Therapy.*

Brecher, Harold and Arline *Forty Something Forever: A Consumer's Guide to Chelation Therapy.*

Cranton, Elmer, M.D. *Bypassing Bypass.*

Rath, Matthias, M.D. *Why Animals Don't Get Heart Attacks...But People Do.*

Rath, Matthias, M.D. *Ten Years That Changed Medicine Forever.*

Hickey, Steve, Ph.D. and Roberts, Hilary, Ph.D. *Ascorbate-The Science of Vitamin C.*

Barnes, Broda, M.D. *Hypothyroidism: The Unsuspected Illness.*

Barnes, Broda, M.D. *Solved: The Riddle of Heart Disease.*

Websites

www.thincs.org The International Network of Cholesterol Skeptics.

www.ravnskov.nu/cholesterol.htm Uffe Ravnskov, M.D.

www.spacedoc.net Duane Graveline, M.D.

www.medicalconsumers.org A non-profit advocacy organization. Some good articles on cholesterol and statins.

www.statinalert.org Much information on statin drug dangers.

www.drugintel.com Shines the light on problems in the pharmaco-medical-industrial complex. Statin risk/benefit article by Joel Kauffman, Ph.D. can be found here.

www.westonaprice.org Lots of free information about traditional foods. Unbiased scientific information about fats, cholesterol, carbohydrates and much more.

www.ICIMED.com International College of Integrative Medicine. Organization of innovative complementary alternative physicians. Physician referral.

www.ACAM.com American College of Advancement in Medicine. Leading organization of alternative physicians, many of whom do chelation therapy. Physician referral.

www.dr-rath-foundation.org Matthias Rath, M.D.

www.paulingtherapy.com Information and a video providing great detail regarding the Pauling-Rath therapy for heart disease.

www.thecureforheartdisease.com Information on the Pauling-Rath therapy for heart disease.

www.brodabarnes.org The Broda Barnes Foundation. Information on thyroid disease and other endocrine problems.

www.vitalchoice.com Source for uncontaminated wild Alaskan salmon, halibut, organic blueberries, and more.

www.eatwild.com Information to help you find natural grass-fed beef, pork, lamb, chicken, turkey in your area.

www.dorway.com Information on aspartame toxicity.

www.wnho.net World Natural Health Organization. Click on "Sweet Misery: A Poisoned World" for information on ordering the DVD that exposes important truths on aspartame.

www.designsforhealth.com A source for top quality nutritional supplements as described in this book. Sold only through health care professionals 800-847-8302.   .

Richard E. Tapert, D.O., C.N.P.
rknew@centurytel.net